World Federation of Neurology
Seminars in Clinical Neurology

STROKE: SELECTED TOPICS

World Federation of Neurology
Seminars in Clinical Neurology

Stroke: Selected Topics

Julien Bogousslavsky, MD, CHAIR
Professor
Department of Neurology
University of Lausanne and
Centre Hospitalier Universitaire Vaudois
Lausanne, Switzerland

Louis R. Caplan, MD
Department of Neurology
Harvard Medical School
Cambridge, Massachusetts
and
Division of Cerebrovascular Disease
Beth Israel Deaconess Medical Center
Boston, Massachusetts

Helen M. Dewey
National Stroke Research Institute
Heidelberg, Australia

Karin Diserens, MD
Department of Neurology
University of Lausanne and
Centre Hospitalier Universitaire Vaudois
Lausanne, Switzerland

Geoffrey A. Donnan. MD, BS, FRACP
National Stroke Research Institute
Heidelberg, Australia

Marco Tulio Medina, MD
Chairman, Neurology Training Program
National Autonomous University of Honduras
Tegucigalpa, Honduras

Gerhard Rothacher, MD
Kliniken Schmieder
Neurological Rehabilitation Hospital
Gailingen, Germany

Luis César Rodríguez Salinas, MD
Department of Neurology
National Autonomous University of Honduras
Tegucigalpa, Honduras

Jonathan Sturm
National Stroke Research Institute
Heidelberg, Australia

Amanda G. Thrift
National Stroke Research Institute
Heidelberg, Australia

Series Editor
Theodore L. Munsat, MD
Professor of Neurology Emeritus
Tufts University School of Medicine
Boston, Massachusetts

New York

Demos Medical Publishing, LLC.
386 Park Avenue South
New York, NY 10016
Visit our website at www.demosmedpub.com

First edition 2006

Library of Congress Cataloging-in-Publication Data

Stroke : selected topics / faculty, Julien Bogousslavsky ... [et al.]. — 1st ed.
      p. ; cm. — (World Federation of Neurology seminars in clinical neurology ; v. 4)
   Includes bibliographical references and index.
   ISBN-13: 978-1-933864-01-3
   ISBN-10: 1-933864-01-X
 1. Cerebrovascular disease. 2. Cerebrovascular disease-—Epidemiology.
   [DNLM: 1. Cerebrovascular Accident. 2. Cerebrovascular
Accident—epidemiology. WL 355 S9213648 2006] I. Bogousslavsky, Julien. II. Series.
   RC388.5.S85658   2006
   616.8'1—dc22
                                                                    2006005408

06 07 08 09 10   5 4 3 2 1
Made in the United States of America

Preface

The recent surveys by the World Health Organization (WHO) have shown that stroke is the second cause of death worldwide, and the first cause of acquired physical disability in adults. In the context of the present increase in ageing populations, the increase of stroke associated with age makes stroke one of the main health issues, the burden of which will markedly continue to develop over the next decades.

On the other hand, while its association with age is significant, stroke also is a rising problem in younger populations, especially in developing and low-resources countries. The ongoing Global Stroke Initiative is a surveillance and prevention project which was initiated at WHO, and is monitored by the International Stroke Society (ISS) with the help of other organizations, including the World Federation of Neurology (WFN). Prevention in at-risk individuals, either before (primary prevention) of after (secondary prevention) a first stroke is indeed the most effective way to reduce the burden of stroke and its medical functional, and social consequences. However, despite effective efforts in prevention, as demonstrated by decreased stroke incidence in countries where such programs have been implemented, acute stroke management remains a major target of modern neurology and medicine for reducing the size and damage of the corresponding brain lesion: stroke units and teams, with specific general and focused therapeutic options starting as soon as possible after the insult have become standard practice in most high-resources areas. However, such acute stroke care possibilities are usually lacking in most less developed countries. Facilitating recovery and neurorehabilitation is the third part of the trial (prevention, acute management, rehabilitation) for fighting stroke and its consequences.

The papers in this issue emphasize some of these critical aspects, underlining the need for global, worldwide, concerted actions against one of the most devastating medical conditions.

Julien Bogousslavsky
University of Lausanne, Switzerland

Editor's Preface

The mission of the World Federation of Neurology (WFN, wfneurology.org) is to develop international programs for the improvement of neurologic health, with an emphasis on developing countries. A major strategic aim is to develop and promote affordable and effective continuing neurologic education for neurologists and related health care providers. With this continuing education series, the WFN has launched a new effort in this direction, with this volume being the fourth course made available. The WFN Seminars in Neurology uses an instructional format that has proven to be successful in controlled trials of educational techniques. Modeled after the American Academy of Neurology's highly successful Continuum, we use proven pedagogical techniques to enhance the effectiveness of the course. These include case-oriented information, key points, multiple choice questions, annotated references, and abundant use of graphic material.

In addition, the course content has a special goal and direction. We live in an economic environment in which even the wealthiest nations have to restrict health care in one form or another. Especially hard pressed are countries where, of necessity, neurologic care is often reduced to the barest essentials or less. There is general agreement that much of this problem is a result of increasing technology. With this in mind, we have asked the faculty to present the instructional material and patient care guidelines with minimal use of expensive technology. Technology of unproven usefulness has not been recommended. However, at the same time, advice on patient care is given without compromising a goal of achieving the very best available care for the patient with neurologic disease. On occasion, details of certain investigative techniques are pulled out of the main text and presented separately for those interested. This approach should be of particular benefit to health care systems that are attempting to provide the best in neurologic care but with limited resources.

These courses are provided to participants by a distribution process unusual for continuing education material. The WFN membership consists of 86 individual national neurologic societies. Societies that have expressed an interest in the program and agree to meet certain specific reporting requirements are provided a limited number of courses without charge. Funding for the program is provided by unrestricted educational grants. Preference is given to neurologic societies with limited resources. Each society receiving material agrees to convene a discussion group of participants at a convenient location within a few months of receiving the material. This discussion group becomes an important component of the learning experience and has proved to be highly successful.

Our fourth course addresses the important area of stroke diagnosis and management. The Chair of this course, Professor Julian Bogousslavsky a recognized international authority, has selected an outstanding faculty of experts. We very much welcome your comments and advice for future courses.

Theodore L. Munsat, M.D.
Professor of Neurology Emeritus
Tufts University School of Medicine
Boston, Massachusetts

Contents

Preface v

Editor's Preface vii

1. The Epidemiology of Stroke 1
   Geoffrey A. Donnan, Helen M. Dewey, Amanda G. Thrift, and Jonathan Sturm

2. Stroke Subtypes and Rationale for Their Separation 9
   Louis R. Caplan

3. Recovery and Rehabilitation 27
   Karin Diserens, Gerhard Rothacher, and Julien Bogousslavsky

4. Stroke in Developing Countries 49
   Luis César Rodriguez Salinas and Marco Tulio Medina

Index 63

CHAPTER 1

THE EPIDEMIOLOGY OF STROKE

Geoffrey A. Donnan, Helen M. Dewey, Amanda G. Thrift, and Jonathan Sturm

KEY POINT

■ In most Western societies, stroke is the third most common cause of death, and it causes significant social and economic burden.

THE BURDEN OF STROKE

In 1990, when the global burden of stroke was assessed by Murray and Lopez as part of the World Bank burden of disease initiative, it was found to be the second most common cause of death after ischemic heart disease (Table 1.1). However, this ranking is somewhat artificial because, if all cancers were grouped together, they would occupy the second rank. Nevertheless, approximately 4.4 million people die from the consequences of stroke each year, totalling about 9% of all deaths. In Western countries, stroke accounts for 10% to 12% of all deaths, and about 88% of these occur in people over the age of 65 years. Expressed in even more immediate terms, for most Western countries, every 8-10th death is due to a stroke,

and the chance of an individual having a stroke increases with age, with the risk doubling every decade over the age of 50 years. In 1990, when the impact of stroke was assessed using disability-adjusted life years (DALYs), the overall burden of stroke ranked as sixth most important behind lower respiratory infections, diarrheal diseases, perinatal disorders, unipolar depression, and ischemic heart disease (see Table 1.1).

Life expectancy has been steadily increasing in most parts of the world, particularly over the last century, largely due to improving economic conditions and health care standards. Because advances in medical care are more readily afforded in developed compared with developing regions, a consequent imbalance in health care expenditure

TABLE 1.1 Ten Leading Causes of Death and DALYs worldwide in 1990

Rank	Cause of Deaths	Number of Deaths (x103)	Disorder	Number of DALYs (x106)
	All causes	50,467		
1	Ischemic heart disease	6,260	Lower respiratory infections	112.9
2	Cerebrovascular disease	4,381	Diarrheal diseases	99.6
3	Lower respiratory infections	4,299	Perinatal disorders	92.3
4	Diarrheal diseases	2,946	Unipolar major depression	50.8
5	Perinatal disorders	2,443	Ischemic heart disease	46.7
6	Chronic obstructive pulmonary disease	2,211	Cerebrovascular disease	38.5
7	Tuberculosis (HIV seropositive excluded)	1,960	Tuberculosis	38.4
8	Measles	1,058	Measles	36.5
9	Road-traffic accidents	999	Road-traffic accidents	34.3
10	Trachea, bronchus, and lung cancers	945	Congenital anomalies	32.9

KEY POINT

■ Fortunately, mortality from stroke has been steadily declining since the 1950s, although it has plateaued more recently.

occurs. Hence, despite the fact that only 7.2% of the burden of disease (as quantitated by DALYs) is carried among the established market economies, these economies consume 87.3% of total health care expenditures. This pattern is almost certainly reflected in expenditures on stroke care. Based on predictions of population increases and life expectancy, it is possible to develop predictive models of the changing burden of disease. By using this approach, Murray and Lopez have estimated that, by the year 2020, stroke will continue to be the second most common cause of death globally. The burden of disability caused by stroke, measured by DALYs, will increase by about 17% from sixth to the second most important contributor in the developed world (Table 1.2). Clearly, these issues must be considered seriously by health care planners in Western countries.

Globally, stroke consumes about 2% to 4% of total health care costs and more than 4% of direct healthcare costs in industrialized countries. The cost of stroke has been estimated using a variety of "bottom-up" and "top-down" approaches in a number of Western countries. An accurate bottom-up costing of stroke was performed by Dewey et al. on the incident cases of the North East Melbourne Stroke Incidence Study (NEMESIS). In that Australian study, the present value of lifetime accrued cost was estimated at $AUD1.3 billion in 1997. In the same year, the total cost estimate for the United States was $US40.9 billion, although these were not incidence-based statistics. Disappointingly, in spite of the magnitude of the problem and the cost to the community, the proportion of research funds directed toward reducing the burden of stroke remains well below most other disease groupings, such as heart disease or cancer, although this pattern appears to be slowly changing.

MORTALITY TRENDS FOR STROKE: REGIONAL DIFFERENCES

Although it is known that death certification is not a precise science and may be prone to decades of fashion influence within and between countries, significant differences do appear to exist in mortality rates for stroke in various parts of the world. The average age-adjusted stroke mortality for Western countries is about 50 to 100 per 100,000 per year and, as mentioned earlier, this accounts for almost 10% to 12% of all deaths. These deaths are best documented among developed nations, where the lowest annual age-adjusted rates recorded from 1989 through to 1992 were in the United States and Canada, while the highest were in Portugal and Czechoslovakia (Figure 1.1). Such marked geographic variations tend to sug-

TABLE 1.2	Ten Projected Leading Causes of DALYs in Developed Regions in 2020	
Rank	Disease or Injury	DALYs (x106)
	All causes	160.5
1	Ischemic heart disease	18.0
2	Cerebrovascular disease	9.9
3	Unipolar major depression	9.8
4	Trachea, bronchus, and lung cancers	7.3
5	Road-traffic accidents	6.9
6	Alcohol use	6.1
7	Osteoarthritis	5.6
8	Dementia and other degenerative and hereditary CNS disorders	5.5
9	Chronic obstructive pulmonary disease	4.9
10	Self-inflicted injuries	3.9

KEY POINT

■ Incidence has been more
difficult to monitor over
the same period, but
appears to trend toward
increases in less well-
developed regions and
reductions in some
developed Western
societies.

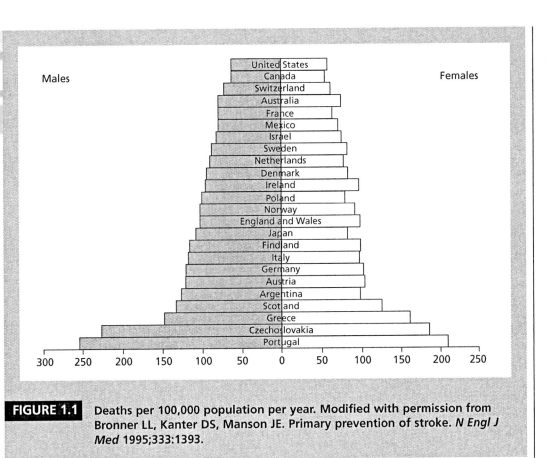

FIGURE 1.1 Deaths per 100,000 population per year. Modified with permission from Bronner LL, Kanter DS, Manson JE. Primary prevention of stroke. *N Engl J Med* 1995;333:1393.

gest an influence of environmental factors on mortality. Differences in risk-factor prevalence as well as management strategies for acute stroke may result in differing case fatality rates.

As mentioned earlier, a constant overall decline in stroke mortality has been noted within the developed world, regardless of regional differences in mortality rates. For example, in Australia, about a 70% decline has occurred since 1950 (Figure 1.2). An average figure for the decline in Western countries is about 1% per year until 1968, and about 5% per year latterly. A number of explanations have been proposed, the most plausible being the steady introduction of blood pressure–lowering agents of increasing efficacy over this period, together with a parallel improvement in living standards—both important risk factors for vascular diseases, including stroke.

MEASURING STROKE INCIDENCE

Of important note, the annual incidence of cerebrovascular events exceeds that of

ischemic heart disease and peripheral vascular disease. One of the main reasons for the majority of incidence studies being carried out in affluent industrialized countries and few, if any, in underdeveloped countries is the expensive and labour-intensive nature of the process. Perhaps, because of this, not all investigators have met the standards required to produce reliable incidence data. Hence, comparisons of stroke incidence data between regions is fraught with difficulty. In response to this problem, a set of criteria for "ideal" incidence studies has been developed so that sensible comparisons could be made between regions in which this benchmark in study standards had been reached. Among these studies, regional differences in incidence do appear to exist among Western countries (Figure 1.3). In Dijon, France, the incidence rates are lowest at about 240 per 100,000 people, standardised to the European population aged 45 to 84 years; whereas in Novosibirsk, Russia, the rates are approximately 600 per 100,000 people. In our own North East Melbourne Stroke

KEY POINT

- Overall, evidence shows an imbalance between mortality and incidence, with declining mortality, but relatively stable incidence. Thus, it is reasonable to assume that, in most countries, prevalence is most likely increasing.

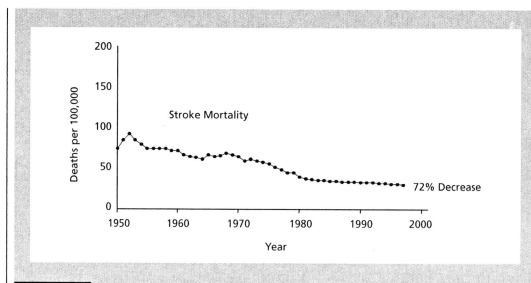

FIGURE 1.2 Age-adjusted death rates 1950–96 in Australia.

Incidence Study (NEMESIS), the incidence was very similar to most developed countries, at 326 per 100,000 people, when adjusted in the same way. As for mortality figures, these regional differences in incidence seem to suggest that environmental and/or genetic factors may play a role.

Longitudinal trends in stroke incidence are even more difficult to ascertain. In Rochester, Minnesota, a steady decline of 45% in incidence occurred from 1945

through 1979, although subarachnoid hemorrhage as a subtype did not change significantly. Among the limited "ideal" incidence studies, even fewer have been repeated years later, and rarely more than once. Most of those repeat studies available that fulfil the ideal criteria are shown in Figure 1.4. As can be seen, a consistent trend does not seem to exist for industrialized nations over the last three decades or so: In four studies, an incidence increase occurred; in one, no

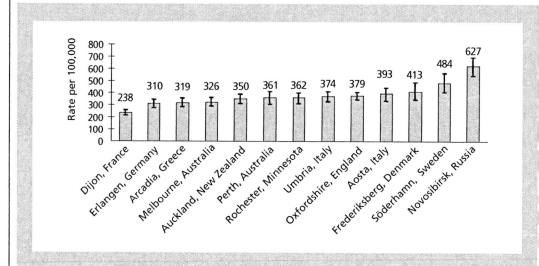

FIGURE 1.3 Comparison of ischemic stroke incidence, standardised to "European" population aged 45 to 84 years.

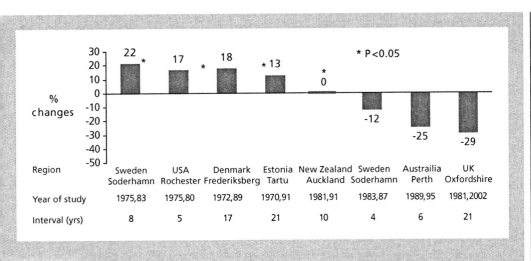

FIGURE 1.4 Ideal stroke incidence studies; change in incidence.

change occurred and, in another, a decline occurred. Interestingly, significant reductions have recently been shown in Perth, Australia, and Oxford, England.

Other data of interest comes from the Monitoring Trends and Determinants in Cardiovascular Disease (MONICA) study. Although not "ideal," particularly given that the age groups studied were only 35 to 69 years and would, therefore, capture only about half of the incident strokes, the methodology was consistent from year to year. A comparison of incidence trends during the years 1987 through 1994 for Northern Sweden (Oktyabrsky and Kirovsky) with those of Novosibirsk in Russia showed a significant increase for the latter but not the former. Again, it seems likely that environmental factors may play a role in these disparate rates.

ESTIMATES OF STROKE PREVALENCE

Despite the obvious advantages of knowing the number of individuals living with the consequences of stroke in a given society, less attention has been paid to stroke prevalence. Several reasons may account for this, the most important being that so few direct measures have been performed. To obtain an accurate "snapshot" of the number of prevalent strokes at a fairly brief period of time, usually by door-to-door survey within a large denominator population, is a daunting task. Typical estimates are in the order of

500 per 100,000 population in industrialized countries (depending on age distribution of each population) and, because of the difficulties mentioned, these estimates often are calculated using incidence and mortality rates, rather than by direct measurement. Because of the inter-relationship between incidence, mortality, and prevalence, longitudinal estimates of prevalence also can be made. Clearly, if mortality is declining in most Western societies, prevalence must be increasing unless, incidence is declining at a similar rate. In Rochester, Minnesota, although 30-day case fatality fell from about 24% during the period 1945–1949 to 12% in 1980–1984, a greater reduction in incidence (45%) was seen during approximately the same period. In Sweden and New Zealand, incidence was unchanged, but case fatality declined. For each of these scenarios, an increase in stroke prevalence and consequent greater burden on the community most likely has occurred. Information such as this is important to enable sensible health care resource planning and allocation.

THE HETEROGENEITY OF STROKE

Stroke is a heterogeneous condition having multiple subtypes, each with a unique mechanism of development and, often, a unique risk factor profile. A distribution of subtypes typical of Western societies was seen in NEMESIS. The major categories were intracerebral hemorrhage (14.5% of all stokes), subarachnoid hemorrhage (4.3%), cerebral infarction (72.5%), and 8.7% of undetermined type. The pathogenesis usually related to small intracerebral vessel rupture, aneurysmal rupture into the subarachnoid space, and vessel occlusion, respectively. Within the ischemic stroke category are further mechanistic subtypes, the most important being lacunar infarction due to in situ small vessel occlusion, large vessel artery to artery embolism and cardioembolic stroke (usually secondary to the presence of atrial fibrillation). A number of well-recognized classification systems of stroke exist, the TOAST system being one of the most commonly used for hospital-based studies, having categories very similar to those described above. The most robust system for use in large community-based epidemiological studies is the Oxfordshire Community Stroke Study classification, because it is only based on clinical findings, without the need for expensive investigations that may not be available in many regions.

RISK FACTORS FOR STROKE

One of the more important contributions of stroke epidemiologists during the latter half of the last century was the identification of the major stroke risk factors. These can be broadly categorized as modifiable or nonmodifiable. Modifiable risk factors such as hypertension, diabetes, and smoking are of more interest to public health planners because of the opportunity available to reduce the burden of stroke by minimizing community exposure. Other risk factors, such as atrial fibrillation and transient ischemic attacks, are of interest because they are somewhat unique to stroke when compared with other vascular diseases. The importance of any given risk factor can be quantitated by *relative risk* and *population-attributable risk*. The former is an index of the importance of the magnitude of the association between those risk-exposed and those who have not been exposed, whereas the latter gives an indication of the proportion of all strokes in the community that could be attributed to a given factor. The prevalence of various risk factors has a major influence on the population-attributable risk. Hence, whereas the relative risk of some factors may be relatively modest, their high prevalence in the community results in a significant population-attributable risk (for example, smoking in many societies).

Interestingly, when all known risk factors for stroke are considered, the total attributable risk only approaches 60%. This suggests that other, yet-to-be-identified risk factors contribute to the remaining 40%. In establishing these as definite risk factors, criteria for causality must be fulfilled. These criteria include the demonstration of an association (increased relative risk), biologic plausibility of the association, a dose–response effect, and demonstration that modification (if possible) of the risk factor will reduce the risk of further stroke events.

STROKE RECURRENCE AND OUTCOME

The development of stroke of any type is associated with an increased risk of recurrence. After an initial stroke, about 20% die within the first 30 days and about 40% by 1 year. Of the survivors, approximately 30% may be disabled and 10% require institutional care. Depression is also a major problem among stroke survivors, with estimates varying between 15% and 30%. Overall, between 6% and 14% will have further stroke in the first year, with the highest rates in the first month. At 5 years, between 20% and 37% will have had a further stroke event, either fatal or nonfatal. Because of the increased chance of repeat stroke, some attention has been paid to understanding risk factors for further events. Surprisingly, factors associated with stroke recurrence are less well documented than for first ever events, but those that emerge consistently are age, hypertension, atrial fibrillation, ischemic heart disease, diabetes, and smoking. Of these, hypertension has been established most rigorously because of the biologic plausibility of its association, a dose–response effect, and reduction of the risk of further stroke events when blood pressure is modified (the PROGRESS study). Atrial fibrillation (nonvalvular) also is well established, although a dose–response effect is less relevant because of its dichotomous pattern.

STROKE PREVENTION

As mentioned earlier, projections concerning the future burden of stroke are a stark reminder that prevention measures must be improved considerably if the absolute numbers of those with stroke are even to remain stable and not increase. Risk factor modification through the combination of an opportunistic and mass community outreach seems to be the most logical approach. It is of interest that the reduction of entire community blood pressures by only 9/5 mm Hg would prevent 20,000 strokes annually in France and 51,000 in the United States. Hence, the mass modification of important risk factors having high attributable risks would seem to be a priority although, in practical terms, the combined approach mentioned maybe the most useful.

REFERENCES

Bamford J, Sandercock P, Dennis M, et al. Classification and natural history of clinically identifiable subtypes of cerebral infarction. *Lancet* 1991;337:1521–26.

Beaglehole R, Bonita R, Kjellstrom T. *Basic epidemiology*. Geneva: World Health Organization, 1993.

Bonita R. Epidemiology of stroke. *Lancet* 1992;339:342.

Bonita R. Stroke trends in Australia and New Zealand: mortality, morbidity, and risk factors. *Ann Epidemiol* 1993;3:529–33.

Broderick JP, Phillips SJ, Whisnant JP, et al. Incidence rates of stroke in the eighties: the end of the decline in stroke? *Stroke* 1989;20:577–82.

Bronner LL, Kanter DS, Manson JE. Primary prevention of stroke. *N Engl J Med* 1995;333:1393.

Burn J, Dennis M, Bamford J, et al. Long-term risk of recurrent stroke after a first-ever stroke. The Oxfordshire Community Stroke Project. *Stroke* 1994;25:333–37.

Dewey HM, Thrift AG, Mihalopoulos C, et al. Cost of stroke in Australia from a societal perspective: Results from the North East Melbourne Stroke Incidence Study (NEMESIS). *Stroke* 2001;32:2409–16.

EAFT (European Atrial Fibrillation Trial) Study Group. Secondary prevention in nonrheumatic atrial fibrillation after transient ischaemic attack or minor stroke. *Lancet* 1993;342:1255–62.

Hardie K, Jamrozik K, Hankey GJ, et al. Trends in five-year survival and risk of recurrent stroke after first-ever stroke in the Perth community stroke study. *Cerebrovasc Dis* 2005;19:179–85.

Harmsen P, Tsipogianni A, Wilhelmsen L. Stroke incidence rates were unchanged, while fatality rates declined, during 1971–1987 in Göteborg, Sweden. *Stroke* 1992;23:1410–15.

Hier DB, Foulkes MA, Swiontoniowski M, et al. Stroke recurrence within 2 yeas after ischemic infarction. *Stroke* 1991;22:155–61.

Hill AB. The environment and disease: Association or causation? *Proc R Soc Med* 1965;58:295–300.

Jamrozik K, Broadhurst RJ, Lai N, et al. Trends in the incidence, severity, and short-term outcome of stroke in Perth, western Australia. *Stroke* 1999;30:2105–11.

Jorgensen HS, Nakayama H, Reith J, et al. Stroke recurrence: predictors, severity, and prognosis. The Copenhagen Stroke Study. *Neurology* 1997;48:891–95.

Meissner I, Whisnant JP, Garraway WM. Hypertension management and stroke recurrence in a community (Rochester, Minnesota, 1950–1979). *Stroke* 1988;19:459–63.

Murray CJL, Lopez AD. Alternative projections of mortality and disability by cause 1990–2020: Global Burden of Disease Study. *Lancet* 1997;349:1498–04.

Murray CJL, Lopez AD. Global mortality, disability, and the contribution of risk factors: Global Burden of Disease Study. *Lancet* 1997;349:1436–42.

Murray CJL, Lopez AD. Mortality by cause for eight regions of the world: Global Burden of Disease Study. *Lancet* 1997;349:1269–76.

PROGRESS Collaborative Group. Randomised trial of a perindopril-based blood pressure lowering regimen among 6,105 patients with prior stroke or transient ischaemic attack. *Lancet* 2001;358:1033–41.

Rothwell PM, Coull AJ, Silver LE, et al., for the Oxford Vascular Study. Population-based study of event-rate, incidence, case fatality, and mortality for all acute vascular events in all arterial territories (Oxford Vascular Study). *Lancet* 2005;366:1773–83.

Rothwell PM, Coull AJ, Giles MF, et al., for the Oxford Vascular Study. Change in stroke incidence, mortality, case-fatality, severity, and risk factors in Oxfordshire, UK from 1981 to 2004 (Oxford Vascular Study). *Lancet* 2004;363:1925–33.

Sacco RL, Wolf PA, Kannel WB, et al. Survival and recurrence following stroke. The Framingham study. *Stroke* 1982;13:290–95.

Stegmayr B, Vinogradova T, Malyutina S, et al. Widening gap of stroke between east and west: eight-year trends in occurrence and risk factors in Russia and Sweden. *Stroke* 2000;31:2–8.

Sudlow CL, Warlow CP. Comparing stroke incidence worldwide: what makes studies comparable? *Stroke* 1996;27:550–58.

Thrift AG, Dewey HM, Macdonell RAL, et al. Stroke incidence on the east coast of Australia: the North East Melbourne Stroke Incidence Study (NEMESIS). *Stroke* 2000;31:2087–92.

Thrift AG, Gilligan AK, Donnan GA. Major risk factors and protective factors: how to improve primary prevention of cerebrovascular disease. In: *Prevention of Ischemic Stroke*, M. Fisher and C. Fieschi, eds. London: Martin Dunitz Publishers Ltd., 2000;7–26.

Whisnant JP. Modelling of risk factors for ischemic stroke: the Willis lecture. *Stroke* 1997;28:1839–43.

CHAPTER 2

STROKE SUBTYPES AND RATIONALE FOR THEIR SEPARATION

Louis R. Caplan

KEY POINT

■ Find out what is wrong with each stroke and cerebrovascular disease patient in as much detail as possible. Even when no proven treatment exists, knowing the details of the condition allows better prognosis and choice of potential treatments.

The two major categories of stroke, hemorrhagic and ischemic, are opposite conditions. In hemorrhage, too much blood is contained within the closed cranial cavity; in ischemia, too little blood is available to meet the oxygen and nutrient need for an area within the brain. Each of these categories can be further subdivided into subtypes, the recognition of which should identify different strategies for treatment.

Intracranial hemorrhage can be divided into intracerebral hemorrhage (ICH) (also called parenchymal hemorrhage), characterized by bleeding directly into brain tissue, and subarachnoid hemorrhage (SAH), characterized by bleeding into the cerebrospinal fluid surrounding the brain and spinal cord. These two subtypes have somewhat different causes, different clinical pictures, different clinical courses, different outcomes, and different treatment strategies.

INTRACRANIAL HEMORRHAGE
Intracerebral Hemorrhage (ICH)
The most common causes of ICH are hypertension, trauma, bleeding diatheses, amyloid angiopathy, illicit drug use (mostly amphetamines and cocaine), and vascular malformations. ICH occasionally is caused by bleeding into tumors and into brain infarcts, aneurysmal rupture, and vasculitis. Hypertension is by far the most common and important cause. Often, the patient had not been hypertensive previously, as in the case of AH in Case 1. A relatively acute increase in blood pressure stresses normal arterioles and causes them to break. Chronic hypertension also can lead to wear and tear on intracerebral arteries and cause hemorrhage. In amyloid angiopathy, the waxy amyloid deposits in the arteries and arterioles makes the arteries more fragile and

CASE 1
A 38-year-old African American man (AH) was moving heavy objects in his garage when he noted a numb feeling in his left arm. He had been in good health, but was overweight. He had no history of hypertension or other vascular disease, but his father and mother both took "high blood pressure pills." He went into the house and, as he walked, he realized that his entire left side, including his limbs, felt numb, and he began to limp. When he reached the house, he could no longer walk and his wife noted that his left face drooped and his voice was slurred. She drove him to the hospital 15 minutes away. During the trip, he complained of headache and began to vomit. Examination in the hospital emergency room showed a blood pressure (BP) of 210/135 mm Hg and a pulse of 70 and regular. AH was drowsy but could easily be aroused. He had a severe left hemiplegia, and his eyes and head were deviated to the right. His left tendon reflexes were increased, and his left plantar response was extensor. Sensation was diminished in his left limbs. A computed tomography (CT) scan showed a moderate-sized hemorrhage in the right basal ganglia-internal capsule region (Figure 2.1).

liable to break. Straining, lifting, and emotional stress can precipitate bleeding.

Bleeding is usually from arterioles or small arteries; hemorrhage is directly into the brain, forming a localized hematoma that spreads along white-matter pathways. An accumulation of blood occurs over minutes to hours; hematomas gradually grow by adding blood at their periphery, like snow-

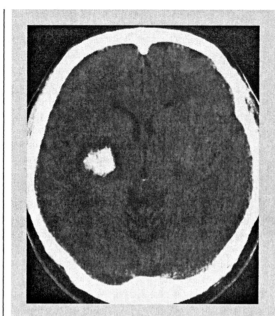 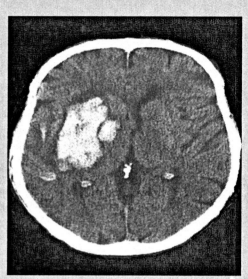

FIGURE 2.1 Small and large basal ganglionic hemorrhages on CT scans.

balls rolling downhill. Hematomas continue to grow until the pressure surrounding them increases enough to limit their spread or until hemorrhages decompress by emptying their contents into the ventricular system or into the cerebrospinal fluid (CSF) on the pial surface of the brain.

The earliest symptoms relate to dysfunction of the portion of the brain that contains the hematoma. Bleeding into the right putamen and internal capsule region, as in AH, causes left limb motor and/or sensory signs, whereas bleeding into the cerebellum causes difficulty in walking, and bleeding into the left temporal lobe presents as aphasia. The neurologic symptoms usually increase gradually during minutes or a few hours. In contrast to brain embolism and SAH, the neurologic symptoms do not begin abruptly and are not maximal at onset. If the hematoma becomes large enough to increase intracranial pressure or cause shifts in intracranial contents, then headache, vomiting, and a decreased level of consciousness develop. In small hemorrhages, these symptoms are absent, and the syndrome is that of a gradually progressing stroke.

ICHs destroy brain tissue as they enlarge. The pressure created by the extra brain contents (blood and surrounding brain edema)

can be life threatening; large hematomas have a high mortality and morbidity. The goal of treatment is to contain and limit the bleeding. Recurrences are unusual if the causative disorder, such as hypertension or bleeding diathesis, is controlled.

Subarachnoid Hemorrhage The most common causes of SAH are rupture of arterial aneurysms that lie at the base of the brain and bleeding from vascular malformations that lie near the pial surface. Bleeding diatheses, trauma, amyloid angiopathy, and illicit drug use are other less common caus-

CASE 2

A 25-year-old woman (BD), during sex with her husband, suddenly complained of severe headache. She looked vacant, and her body went limp. Moments later, she became responsive but appeared dazed. She began to vomit. In the hospital emergency room, she was very drowsy and difficult to arouse. Her BP was 130/60. Her neck was stiff, and her plantar responses were extensor. She had no asymmetric abnormalities of vision, movement, or feeling. A CT scan showed extensive subarachnoid blood (Figure 2.2). Angiography later showed a middle cerebral artery aneurysm.

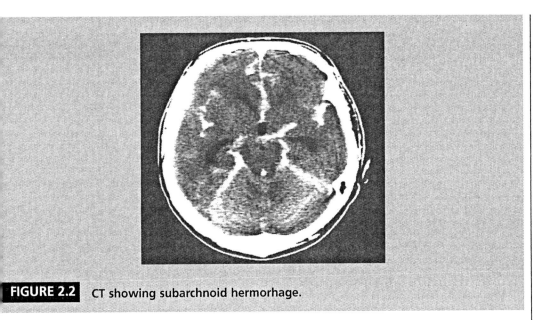

FIGURE 2.2 CT showing subarchnoid hermorhage.

es. Rupture of an aneurysm releases blood directly into the CSF under arterial pressure. The blood spreads quickly within the CSF, rapidly increasing intracranial pressure. If bleeding continues, death or deep coma ensues. Usually, the bleeding is only for a few seconds. Aneurysmal rupture can be triggered by strain, sex, or physical effort, as in BD, in Case 2. Rebleeding is very common. In patients with nonaneurysmal SAH, the bleeding is less abrupt and may develop over a longer period of time.

The symptoms in patients with aneurysmal SAH begin abruptly. The sudden increase in pressure causes a cessation of activity, often loss of memory or focus, knees buckling, and the like. Headache is an invariable symptom, and is usually instantly severe and widespread. Headache may radiate into the neck or even down the back into the legs. Vomiting occurs soon after onset. Usually, no important focal neurologic signs occur unless bleeding occurs both into the brain and into the CSF at the same time (meningeo-cerebral hemorrhage).

The aim of treatment is to identify the cause and quickly treat it to prevent rebleeding. The other goal of treatment is to prevent brain damage due to delayed ischemia related to vasoconstriction of intracranial arteries. Blood within the CSF induces vasoconstriction that can be intense and severe and lead to underperfusion of brain tissue.

BRAIN ISCHEMIA

Three main subtypes of brain ischemia exist: thrombosis, embolism, and systemic hypoperfusion. Embolism refers to passage of materials, most often thrombi, from the place where they developed into a distant location in the vascular bed. *Thrombosis* is a term usually restricted to the in situ development of occlusive lesions. The most common cause is atherosclerosis, and occlusive thrombi may be superimposed on atherosclerotic plaques. Systemic hypoperfusion refers to a general decrease in cerebral blood flow, most often related to hypotension, hypoxia, and decreased blood volume.

A plumbing analogy helps explain to patients the difference and importance of these ischemic subdivisions. Suppose a faucet in the bathroom on the third floor of your house doesn't work—water dribbles out. You call a plumber. The problem could be rust and blockage of a large pipe that leads directly to that sink. If so, the plumber could repair the situation by fixing that pipe. That situation is analogous to *thrombosis*, a term used to indicate a local in situ obstruction of an artery. Or, the obstruction could be due to disease of the arterial wall such as arteriosclerosis, dissection, fibromuscular dysplasia, and superimposed thrombosis may or may not be present. The process is a local one that might involve a large extracranial or intracranial artery or a penetrating artery.

Suppose, instead, that a piece of debris had gotten into the water system and blocked the pipe to that sink. Then, repairing the pipe would help temporarily, but if the source of the debris were not identified and removed, further pipes would become blocked. This situation is akin to *embolism*, in which particles originating elsewhere block arterial blood supply to a brain region. A third possibility would be a general malfunction of the plumbing system—lack of water in the tank, low water pressure, or something similar. Then, the problem would not be in any one pipe, but attention would be directed to the central water delivery apparatus. This situation is akin to *systemic hypoperfusion*, a more general circulatory problem manifesting itself in the brain. Like the third-floor sink, the brain is the highest place above the heart to which the heart must pump blood; it is also the most vulnerable to a deficiency of blood flow. Separating these mechanisms is critical for the success of the plumber and for the physician who cares for patients with brain ischemia.

Thrombosis Atherosclerosis is by far the most common cause of in situ local disease within the large extracranial and intracranial arteries that supply the brain. In patients with hypercoagulable states, white platelet fibrin and red erythrocyte-fibrin thrombi are often superimposed on atherosclerotic lesions or may develop without severe vascular disease. Vasoconstriction, as occurs for example in migraine, is likely the next most common condition, followed in frequency by arterial dissections (a disorder much more common than previously recog-

nized) and traumatic occlusions Fibromuscular dysplasia is an uncommon arteriopathy. Although arteritis is frequently mentioned in the differential diagnosis, its occurrence as a cause of stroke is extremely rare. It is probably considered 1,000 times for each instance that it actually occurs.

Turning to the smaller arteries and arterioles that penetrate at right angles to supply the deeper structures within the brain (basal ganglia, internal capsule, thalamus, pons etc.), the most common cause of obstruction is *lipohyalinosis*, the blockage of an artery by medial hypertrophy and lipid admixed with fibrinoid material in the hypertrophied arterial wall. Lipohyalinosis most often is caused by hypertension but aging also likely plays a role. Micro-atheromas also can block these small penetrating arteries, as can plaques within the larger arteries, which block or extend into the orifices of the branches (called *atheromatous branch disease*). These two subtypes of thrombosis—large artery disease and penetrating artery disease—are worth separating, because the causes, outcomes, and treatments are different.

Because treatment of a local problem can be local (surgery, angioplasty, intra-arterial thrombolysis), identification of the focal vascular lesion (including its nature, severity, and localization) is important for treatment. It should be possible clinically in most patients to determine whether the local vascular disease is within the anterior (carotid) or posterior (vertebrobasilar) circulation and whether the disorder affects large arteries or penetrators.

CASE 3
A 66-year-old white man (SD), one morning noted weakness and numbness of his left arm and hand. He had been taking antihypertensive medicines for 10 years. He smoked a pack of cigarettes each day. Two years previously, he had had a myocardial infarct. When he walked several blocks, he developed pain in his left calf, a symptom that he had not shared with his doctor. Three weeks ago, he had his first attack of weakness of the left hand. This lasted just 2 minutes, and he recovered. Since then, he has had three other brief attacks : In one, the left leg was weak; in another, the left arm and leg felt weak and numb and, during the third attack, his left face felt tingly. Ten days ago, he noted a dark shade descending over the vision in his right eye, a symptom that lasted only 1 minute. When he reached his doctor's office, his arm and hand were normal, and he had no abnormal neurologic signs. A CT scan showed a small infarct in the right parietal lobe. Duplex ultrasound showed an occlusion of his left internal carotid artery in the neck.

The delivery of adequate blood through a blocked or partially blocked artery depends on many factors including blood pressure, blood viscosity, collateral blood flow, and the like. Also, local vascular lesions often are the source of emboli that break off, and these may block distal arteries either transiently or long enough to cause brain infarction. Neurologic symptoms are due to hypoperfusion and/or embolism. In patients with thrombosis, the neurologic symptoms often fluctuate, remit, or progress in a gradual, stuttering, or stepwise fashion.

Embolism   Three main components make up a brain embolism—the donor source (heart, aorta, systemic veins through a cardiac or intrapulmonary defect, and proximal arterial system), the embolic material (the "stuff" that embolizes), and the recipient site. Remember that the recipient site can't tell where the stuff comes from or what it is. The symptoms are neurologic and depend on the region of brain rendered ischemic. The stuff suddenly blocks the recipient site so that the onset is abrupt and usually maximal at onset. Unlike thrombosis, multiple recipient sites within different vascular territories may be present. Infarcts usually are larger than those associated with a local in situ thrombotic etiology. The most common recipient sites of emboli are the middle cerebral arteries, the intracranial ver-

tebral artery and its posterior inferior cerebellar artery branch, and the rostral basilar artery and its superior cerebellar and posterior cerebral artery branches. Treatment depends on the nature of the "stuff" and the source whence it came.

Systemic Hypoperfusion   In this brain ischemia subtype, diminished blood flow is more global and does not affect isolated regions. Reduced perfusion can be attributed to cardiac pump failure caused by cardiac arrest, arrhythmia, or reduced cardiac output related to acute myocardial ischemia, pulmonary embolism, or a pericardial effusion. Hypoxemia can be a complicating factor that reduces the amount of oxygen carried by the blood to the brain. Hypovolemia due to bleeding or other causes of reduced blood volume can also cause hypotension and systemic hypoperfusion.

Characteristically, symptoms of brain dysfunction are diffuse and nonfocal in contrast to the other two categories of ischemia, thrombosis and embolism, in which the signs are focal. Usually, other evidence is present of circulatory compromise and hypotension. Pallor, sweating, tachycardia or severe bradycardia, and low blood pressure usually are present. Neurologic signs are usually bilateral and may indicate involvement of border-zone regions between the major cerebral supply arteries because these areas are most vulnerable to systemic hypoperfusion. These signs include cortical blindness or at least bilateral visual loss, stupor, and weakness of the shoulders and thighs with sparing of the face, hands, and feet (a pattern likened to a "man-in-a-barrel"). Occasionally, the neurologic signs are asymmetric when preexistent asymmetrical cranio-cerebral vascular occlusive disease is present.

CASE 4

A 68-year-old man (HR) suddenly became speechless and fell from his chair. He had had coronary artery bypass surgery 1 year before, and he had a long history of hypertension and hypercholesterolemia. When examined in the hospital, he had a severe right hemiplegia and was mute. A CT scan showed a large infarct involving the deep and superficial portions of the left middle cerebral artery. Neck duplex examination showed only minimal plaques in the carotid arteries. Transesophageal echocardiography showed a large mobile pedunculated plaque, 6 mm in size, in the aortic arch. No thrombi or potentially embolic sources were present in the heart.

CASE 5

A 55-year-old man with known angina pectoris suddenly slumps to the floor. Emergency paramedics find him pulseless and resuscitate him. When he arrives at the hospital, his pulse is 75 and blood pressure is 100/80. He is comatose, but has normal pupillary, corneal, and oculovestibular reflexes. Plantar responses are extensor.

KEY POINT

- Proceed with a sequential diagnosis: First consider stroke mimics. If a stroke, separate hemorrhage from ischemia. If a hemorrhage, separate subarachnoid from intracerebral bleeding. If ischemic, separate thromboembolism from systemic hypoperfusion.

TRANSIENT ISCHEMIC ATTACKS

Recall that SD (Case 3), a patient who had an internal carotid artery occlusion, had had temporary attacks of limb and eye ischemia. One of the typical presentations of cerebrovascular disease is one or more temporary episodes usually labelled as TIAs. TIAs are transient attacks of focal brain ischemia that usually last less than an hour. Most TIAs last less than 5 minutes. TIAs are caused by decreased blood flow to a local portion of the brain; this reduction in flow is related to blockage of blood flow to a brain region due to in situ occlusion of a supply artery or to embolism to that artery. Symptoms are focal, meaning that they relate to dysfunction of a localized part of the brain. Symptoms are transient when the arterial blockage passes (for example dissolution or distal passage of an embolus) or when collateral circulation is able to restore adequate perfusion to the region of ischemia. The symptoms and signs may fluctuate depending on the adequacy of perfusion. Perfusion depends on systemic factors (blood volume, cardiac output, blood pressure, blood viscosity) and local factors (propagation and embolization of clot, development of collateral circulation).

Transient brain ischemia can be caused by a variety of very different conditions. Brain embolism arising from the heart, aorta, or proximal arteries can cause transient attacks of central nervous system dysfunction with good recovery. Occlusive lesions of either large extracranial or intracranial arteries produce transient ischemia by intermittent hypoperfusion of the symptomatic regions of the brain, or by embolization of fibrin-platelet (white thrombi) or erythrocyte-fibrin (red thrombi) clots into the distal brain circulation. Emboli often break up or pass through the vasculature, thus explaining the transiency of the neurologic symptoms. Transient ischemia also occurs in patients with occlusive lesions, either lipohyalinosis or atheromatous branch disease, of the small microscopic-sized intracranial arteries and arterioles. Hypercoagulability and diseases that cause thrombosis of small vessels, such as thrombotic thrombocytopenic purpura, can also cause transient neurologic ischemic symptoms.

THE CLINICAL ENCOUNTER: HISTORY AND EXAMINATION

Features of the history and examination help diagnose these different stroke mechanisms and subtypes.

The Clinical History

Ecology and Risk Factors Demographic and historical features provide probabilities of the patient having one or more of the stroke subtypes. Age, sex, and race are important demographic variables known to clinicians even before they take a history. Most thrombotic and embolic strokes related to atherosclerosis occur in older patients. Individuals under 40 rarely have severe atherosclerosis unless they also have important risk factors such as diabetes, hypertension, hyperlipidemia, smoking, strong family history, etc. On the other hand, hemorrhages, both ICH and SAH, are common in adolescents and young adults. Cardiac-origin embolism also is common in young people with heart disease. Hypertensive ICH is more common among blacks and individuals of Asian descent than among whites. Premenopausal women have a lower frequency of atherosclerosis than men of similar age, unless they have major stroke risk factors. Blacks, Asians, and women have a lower incidence of occlusive disease of the extracranial carotid and vertebral arteries than white men.

Hypertension is the most common and most important stroke risk factor. Severe uncontrolled hypertension is a very strong risk factor for ICH. A young person who enters the hospital with the acute onset of a focal neurologic deficit and who has a blood pressure greater than 220/120 mm Hg has a very high likelihood of having an ICH. Chronic hypertension is a risk factor for both thrombotic extracranial and intracranial large artery disease and penetrating artery disease. The systolic blood pressure is as important or more important than the diastolic pressure. The absence of a history of hypertension or of present hypertension reduces the likelihood of ICH and penetrating artery disease.

Smoking increases the likelihood of extracranial occlusive vascular disease. Diabetes increases the likelihood of large and small artery occlusive disease, but does not predispose to hemorrhage. The use of amphetamines increases the likelihood of both ICH and SAH, but not brain ischemia. Cocaine-related strokes are often hemorrhagic (ICH and SAH), and these hemorrhages often are related to aneurysms and vascular malformations. Cocaine also is associated with brain ischemia, especially involving the posterior circulation's intracranial arteries, and likely is due to vasoconstriction. Cardiac valvular disease, prior myocardial infarction, atrial fibrillation, and endocarditis clearly increase the probability of a stroke being due to embolism. Stroke during the puerperium or in patients taking oral contraceptives (especially high dose) has an increased likelihood of being related to venous or arterial thrombosis. The presence of a known bleeding disorder or prescription of warfarin or other anticoagulants predisposes to hemorrhage either into the brain or into the CSF.

Preexisting conditions affect the likelihood of the presence of one or more of the stroke subtypes. Some conditions (for example, hypertension) predispose to more than one subtype (thrombosis, ICH). The presence of a previous myocardial infarct increases the likelihood of cardiac-origin embolism, but also increases the likelihood of carotid and vertebral artery neck occlusive disease (thrombosis), because atherosclerotic disease of the coronary and extracranial arteries often coexist. A clinician cannot make a firm diagnosis simply on the basis of probability. An older patient with severe atherosclerosis could also harbor an unexpected cerebral aneurysm.

Clinical Course The single most helpful historical item in separating stroke subtypes is the pace and course of the development of symptoms and signs and their clearing—the course of illness. Each stroke subtype has a characteristic time course. Thrombosis-related symptoms often fluctuate, vary between normal and abnormal, or progress in a gradual, stepwise, or stuttering manner, with some periods of improvement. Penetrating artery occlusions usually cause symptoms that develop during a short period of time—usually hours or at most a few days, whereas large artery-related brain ischemia can evolve over a longer period. Patients with ICHs do not improve during the early period but worsen gradually during

minutes or a few hours. Embolic strokes most often occur suddenly, and the deficits indicate focal loss of brain function that is usually (more than 80% of the time) maximal at onset. Rapid recovery also favors embolism. Similarly, aneurysmal SAH develops in an instant, and the symptoms (headache, vomiting, decreased alertness) are due to increased intracranial pressure and blood in the CSF; focal brain dysfunction is less common.

Patients often are unsophisticated and have not monitored their own neurologic functions. Physicians should adopt a strategy called "walking through the events in detail." Could the patient walk, talk, use the phone, use the hand, as the events developed after the first symptoms?

Transient Ischemic Attacks The presence of TIAs, especially more than one, in the same vascular territory as the stroke strongly favors the presence of a local vascular lesion (thrombosis) involving the artery supplying the zone related to the brain ischemia. Attacks in more than one vascular territory suggests brain embolism from the heart or aorta. TIAs are not a feature of brain hemorrhage, although minor hemorrhages manifested by headaches—so-called sentinel hemorrhages—may precede a more major SAH.

Many patients are naive about their nervous systems. They may not volunteer that a week before the stroke that involved their left leg, their left hand became temporarily weak for 10 minutes, or that 2 weeks before, they noted a temporary gray shade that blocked vision in the right eye for about 3 minutes. Many patients would not relate the hand and eye symptoms to the leg symptoms. Physicians must ask directly about specific symptoms—Did your arm, hand, or leg ever go numb? Did you ever have difficulty speaking? Did you ever lose vision? If so, in which part of your vision? Was it in one eye and if so, which one?

Activity at the Onset or Just Before the Stroke Hemorrhages (ICH and SAH) can be precipitated by sex or other physical activity, whereas thrombotic strokes are unusual under those circumstances. Trauma before the stroke suggests traumatic dissection of arteries or traumatic brain hemorrhage. Sudden coughing and sneezing sometimes precipitates brain embolism. Similarly, getting up during the night to urinate seems to promote brain embolism.

Accompanying Symptoms Symptoms unrelated to loss of brain functions, such as fever, headache, vomiting, seizures, and hypotension also can suggest stroke subtype. Fever raises the suspicion of endocarditis. Infections also activate acute phase blood reactants and so also predispose to thrombosis. Severe headache at onset favors SAH, whereas headache that develops after onset and is accompanied by gradually increasing neurologic signs, decreased consciousness, and vomiting is most often indicative of ICH. Some patients have headaches during the days and weeks before thrombotic strokes. Past intermittent severe headaches that are instantaneous at onset, last days, and prevent daily activities often reflect the presence of an aneurysm. These headaches often are caused by small bleeds—so-called "sentinel leaks." Vomiting is common in patients with ICH, SAH, and posterior circulation large artery disease–related ischemia. Seizures are most common in patients with lobar ICHs and in patients with brain emboli, Seizures are rare in patients with acute thrombosis. Reduced alertness favors the presence of hemorrhage—ICH if accompanied by focal neurologic signs and SAH if no important focal signs are present. Loss of consciousness is common in patients with large embolic strokes and in thrombotic and embolic strokes that involve the posterior circulation large arteries.

Findings during the General Physical Examination Clues to stroke subtype can also be found during the general examination. The blood pressure is of obvious importance. Absent pulses (inferior extremity, radial, or carotid) favor atherosclerosis with thrombosis, although the sudden onset of a cold, blue limb favors embolism. Although the internal carotid arteries in the neck cannot be reliably palpated, in some patients occlusion of the common carotid artery in the neck can be diagnosed by the absence of a carotid pulse. An audible neck bruit suggests the presence of occlusive extracranial disease, especially if the bruit is long, focal,

and high-pitched. Palpating the facial pulses is helpful in diagnosing common carotid and internal carotid artery occlusions and temporal arteritis. In common carotid artery occlusions, the facial pulses on the side of the occlusion often are lost. In some patients with internal carotid artery occlusion, the facial pulses are increased on the side of the occlusion because collateral channels often develop between the external carotid artery facial branches and the carotid arteries intracranially.

Abnormalities found on examining the heart, especially murmurs, an irregularly irregular rhythm, and cardiac enlargement, favor cardiac-origin embolism. Similarly, very slow and very fast pulses suggest embolism, especially if the pulse is irregular. Careful ophthalmoscopic examination can uncover the presence of cholesterol crystal, white platelet-fibrin, and red clot emboli. Subhyaloid hemorrhages in the eye (bleeds with a fluid level) suggest a suddenly developing ICH or subarachnoid hemorrhage. When the carotid artery is occluded, the iris may appear speckled, and the ipsilateral pupil may become dilated and poorly reactive. In that circumstance, the retina may also show evidence of chronic ischemia (so-called venous stasis retinopathy).

Neurologic Findings The patient's account of his neurologic symptoms and the neurologic signs found on examination tell more about where the process is in the brain rather than what the lesion is (stroke subtype). Sometimes the presence of some groups of symptoms and signs suggests a specific process, for example, weakness of the face, arm, and leg on one side of the body unaccompanied by sensory, visual, or cognitive abnormalities (so-called pure motor stroke) favors a thrombotic stroke involving penetrating arteries or a small ICH. Large focal neurologic deficits that begin abruptly or progress quickly are characteristic of embolism or ICH.

The presence of some symptoms and signs suggests involvement of the posterior circulation; these include vertigo, staggering, diplopia, deafness, crossed (one side of the face and other side of the body) or bilateral motor and/or sensory signs, and hemianopia. Abnormalities of language suggests anterior circulation disease, as does the presence of motor and sensory signs that parallel each other in their involvement (for example, weakness and numbness of the hand and face on one side).

Although many of these historical and examination features suggest certain stroke subtypes, precise diagnosis cannot be accurately and precisely determined without brain and vascular imaging testing.

LOCATIONS OF VASCULAR PATHOLOGIES

Knowledge of the usual brain and vascular locations and appearances of the various stroke subtypes and pathologies is important for their recognition.

Thrombosis Atherosclerotic narrowing in the anterior circulation most often develops at the origins of the ICAs in the neck. The remainder of the nuchal ICAs are seldom affected, but the carotid siphon is a frequent site for atheromas. The supraclinoid carotid arteries and the main-stem MCAs and ACAs are affected less often than the neck and siphon portions of the ICAs in white men, although in black, Chinese, and Japanese patients, MCA disease is more common than disease of the ICAs. Atherosclerotic narrowing in the posterior circulation is found most often at the proximal origins of the vertebral arteries (VAs) and the subclavian arteries, the proximal and distal ends of the intracranial vertebral arteries, the basilar artery, and the proximal portions of the posterior cerebral arteries (PCAs). Atherosclerotic narrowing rarely affects the distal superficial branches of the cerebral and cerebellar arteries.

Lipohyalinosis and medial hypertrophy secondary to hypertension affect mostly the penetrating lenticulostriate branches of the MCAs, the anterior perforating vessels of the anterior cerebral arteries (ACAs), penetrating arteries originating from the anterior choroidal arteries (AChAs), the thalamogeniculate penetrators from the PCAs, and the paramedian perforating vessels to the pons, midbrain, and thalamus from the basilar artery. Atheromatous plaques within parent arteries and microatheromas within the orifices of branches also can block flow in penetrating arteries. The distribution of

atheromatous branch disease is the same as that of lipohyalinosis, except that atheromatous branch disease may also obstruct larger branches (e.g., the anterior choroidal artery branches of the ICAs and the thalamogeniculate pedicles from the PCAs).

Dissection—traumatic or spontaneous tearing of a vessel wall with intramural bleeding—usually involves the distal extracranial carotid and vertebral arteries. Less common are dissections of the intracranial ICAs, MCAs, VAs, and basilar arteries. Temporal arteritis characteristically affects the ICAs and VAs just before they pierce the dura to enter the cranial cavity, as well as branches of the ophthalmic arteries before they pierce the globe.

Embolism Emboli can block any artery, depending on the size and nature of the embolic material. Large emboli, often clots formed within the heart, can block even large extracranial arteries, such as the innominate, subclavian, carotid, and vertebral arteries in the neck. More often, smaller thrombi formed in the heart, aorta, or the proximal arteries embolize to block intracranial arteries, such as the ICAs, MCAs, ACAs, VAs, basilar artery, and PCAs. Within the anterior circulation, a strong predilection exists for emboli to go to the MCAs and their branches. Within the posterior circulation, thrombi preferentially block the intracranial VAs, the distal basilar artery, the superior cerebellar arteries (SCAs), and the PCAs. Smaller fragments—such as tiny or fragmented thrombi, platelet-fibrin clumps, cholesterol crystals and other fragments from atheromatous plaques, and calcified fragments from valve and vessel surfaces—tend to embolize to superficial small branches of the cerebral and cerebellar arteries and the ophthalmic and retinal arteries.

Intracerebral Hemorrhage Intracerebral hemorrhage is often caused by hypertensive damage to small penetrating vessels, and has the same vascular distribution as lipohyalinosis. The most frequent sites are the striato-capsular region, caudate nucleus, thalamus, pons, and cerebellum. Sudden increases in blood pressure and blood flow can also cause these same penetrating arteries to break, even in the absence of chronic hypertensive changes. Vascular malformations (arteriovenous malformations and cavernous angiomas) can occur anywhere within the brain and lead to intra-parenchymatous bleeding.

Subarachnoid Hemorrhage Aneurysms most often affect junctional regions of the larger vessels of the circle of Willis. The ICA-posterior-communicating-artery junction, anterior communicating artery-ACA junction, and the MCA bifurcations are the most common sites. The supraclinoid ICAs, pericallosal arteries, vertebral-PICA junctions, and apex of the basilar artery also are frequent locations. Vascular malformations that cause the syndrome of subarachnoid hemorrhage are located either in the brain, abutting on pial or ventricular surfaces, or situated within the ventricular system or the subarachnoid space. Some malformations are located entirely within the subarachnoid cerebrospinal fluid compartment.

DIAGNOSIS

Diagnosis should proceed logically and thoughtfully. First, consider whether the process is due to cerebrovascular disease stroke or some other pathology. If the patient has a stroke, is it a hemorrhagic or an ischemic stroke? If a hemorrhagic stroke, is it subarachnoid or intraparenchymatous? If the process is ischemic, is it thrombotic, embolic, or due to systemic hypoperfusion? What, where, and how severe are the causative vascular lesions?

Next, consider whether the symptoms might be due to nonvascular disorders.

TIAs are by definition temporary spells of focal brain dysfunction. The differential diagnosis includes all other causes of transient spells. The four most important and frequent causes of discrete self-limited attacks are seizures (fits), transient ischemic attacks (TIAs), migraine auras, and syncope (faints). Less frequent causes include pressure- or position-related peripheral nerve or nerve root compression that causes transient paresthesias and numbness; peripheral vestibulopathies that cause transient episodic dizziness; and metabolic perturbations such as hypoglycemia, liver, renal, and pulmonary encephalopathies, which can produce episodic abnormal behavior and movements. Patients with brain tumors also occa-

sionally have transient attacks of worsening (so-called "tumor attacks"); the mechanism of the transient neurologic symptoms and signs in tumor patients is thought to be caused by mechanical changes that cause pressure on structures adjacent to the tumor. Similarly, patients with subdural hematomas may have attacks of transient neurologic dysfunction probably related to pressure on adjacent brain tissue. Multiple sclerosis occasionally also can cause brief, recurrent paroxysmal attacks, especially of ataxia and dysarthria. Patients with hysteria and other psychiatric disorders have attacks that include swoons, falls, and episodic blindness, deafness, paralysis, and the like that can be confused with organic loss of function. Transient global amnesia (TGA) is a syndrome characterized by the temporary inability to make new memories, accompanied by retrograde amnesia, which is of uncertain cause but usually is not caused by seizures or transient ischemia.

Features Distinguishing the Cause of Transient Attacks Some disorders cause focal abnormalities of brain function, whereas others cause dysfunction that is either widespread or difficult to localize to any one anatomic region. Some disorders can cause both focal and nonfocal attacks. Seizures, for example, can begin or remain focal, or can be generalized. Similarly, patients with hypoglycemia usually have global deficits in alertness and cognition but occasionally have focal symptoms, such as hemiplegia. Table 2.1 lists the common and less common causes of attacks and their relative tendency to cause focal and nonfocal symptoms.

Other important features of attacks helpful in differential diagnosis include the nature of the symptoms and their progression, duration and timing, and accompanying symptoms that occur during and after the attacks. Table 2.2 shows features that help separate the four most common causes of transient spells. Symptoms can be categorized using Jacksonian terminology as either "positive" or "negative." Positive symptoms indicate active discharge from central nervous system neurons. Typical "positive" symptoms can be visual—bright lines, shapes, objects; auditory—tinnitus, noises, music; somatosensory—burning,

TABLE 2.1 Causes of Transient Attacks and Their Tendency to Cause Focal or Nonfocal Symptoms

Conditions	Focal Symptoms	Nonfocal Symptoms
Common disorders		
Seizures	++	++
TIAs	++++	occasionally
Migraine	++++	
Syncope		++++
Less common disorders		
Vestibulopathy	++	++
Metabolic	+	+++
"Tumor attachks"	+++	+
Multiple sclerosis	++++	
Psychiatric	++	++
Nerves and nerve root	++++	
TGA	++++	

pain, paresthesias; and motor—jerking or repetitive rhythmic movements. In contrast, "negative" symptoms indicate an absence or loss of function: loss of vision, hearing, feeling, or ability to move a part of the body. Seizures and migraine auras characteristical-

TABLE 2.2 Differential Diagnostic Features of TIAs

	Seizures	TIAs	Migraine	Syncope
Demography	Any age Youths are most common	Older patients; Stroke risk factors present; Men > women	Younger age women > men	Any age often younger women > men
CNS Symptoms	Positivesymptoms: limb jerking, head turning; loss of consciousness; negative symptoms may develop and remain postictally and persist	Negative symptoms: numbness visual loss paralysis ataxia; all sensory modalities affected simultaneously	First positive symptomst then negative in same modality; scintillating scotomas and paresthesias most common; 2nd sensory modality is involved after the first clears	Light-headed, dim vision, noises distant, decreased alertness; transient loss of consciousness
Timing	20–180 sec ; absence,atonic seizures and myoclonic jerks are shorter; postictal depression; spells occur during years	Usually minutes; Mostly < 1 hr; spells during days, weeks, or months not usually years	Usually 20–30 minutes; sporadic attacks during years	Usually a few seconds; sporadic attacks during years
Associated symptoms	Tongue biting, incontinence, muscles sore, headache after attack	Headaches may occur during time period of the TIAs	Headache after; nausea. vomiting photophobia phonophobia	Sweating pallor nausea

ly (but not always) begin with positive symptoms, whereas TIAs most often are characterized by "negative" symptoms. Seizures occasionally cause paralytic attacks, but on close observation features of the history and examination usually are present to suggest the presence of seizure discharge. Minor twitching of a finger or toe are common.

The progression and course of the symptoms are helpful in differential diagnosis. Migrainous accompaniments (auras) often progress slowly within one sensory modality. Scintillations or bright objects tend to move slowly across the visual field. Paresthesias may gradually progress from one finger to all the digits, to the wrist, forearm, shoulder, trunk, and then the face and leg. Usually, progression occurs over the course of minutes. After the positive symptoms move, they often are followed by loss of function. The moving train of visual scintillations may leave in its wake a scotoma or visual field defect. As the paresthesias travel centripetally, they may leave the initial areas of skin numb and devoid of feeling. In migrainous auras, symptoms often progress from one modality to another. After the visual symptoms clear, then paresthesias begin. When paresthesias clear, then aphasia or other cortical function abnormalities may develop.

In contrast to migraine, seizures usually (but not always) consist of positive phenomena, most often in one modality, that progress very quickly during seconds. In TIAs, the symptoms are negative; when more than one modality or function is involved, all are affected at about the same time. Loss of consciousness is very common in seizures and syncope, but extremely rare in TIAs. Seizures and syncope usually produce relatively stereotyped attacks, whereas symptoms can be stereotyped or different in various TIAs.

The duration and tempo of attacks also are useful in predicting cause. Migrainous auras characteristically last 20 to 30 minutes, but can last hours. TIAs usually are very fleeting, but in the great majority of patients last less than 1 hour. Seizures last on average about 30 seconds to 3 minutes. Some seizures, including absence attacks, atonic seizures, and myoclonic jerks, are shorter in duration. Syncope is very brief (seconds) unless the patient is artificially propped up or otherwise cannot obtain a supine position. Seizures occur sporadically over the course of years, but sometimes appear in flurries. TIAs usually cluster during a finite period of time. Syncopal attacks are scattered over years. Attacks distributed randomly over many years are almost always either faints, migraine, or seizures. TIAs almost never continue over a span of many years.

Precipitants often give clues to the cause of attacks. Activation of seizures is well known to occur in some patients after stroboscopic stimulation, hyperventilation, reading, or other stimuli. Cessation of anticonvulsants, fever, and alcohol and drug withdrawal are all well known to precipitate seizures in susceptible individuals. In some patients, TIAs occur when blood pressure is reduced, or on sudden standing or bending. Dizziness and vertigo in patients with peripheral vestibulopathies often occur after sudden movements and positional changes. Syncope often occurs when patients see blood, have or are about to have blood drawn or undergo other medical procedures, see an electric saw poised to remove a plaster cast on their arm or leg, stand up for a long time in church, or when a dental drill is aimed directly at their open mouth by a dentist. Hypovolemia also often precipitates faints.

Non-neurologic accompanying symptoms give many attacks a characteristic signature. Headaches are common after migraine auras and after seizures. Headache may occur during the time period of the TIAs, but rarely occur at the same time or directly after neurologic symptoms. A bitten tongue, incontinence, and muscle aches are frequent aftereffects of seizures. Vomiting is common after migraine, and occasionally follows syncope but must be extremely rare after or during TIAs and in relation to seizures. Ictal epileptic vomiting occurs, but is very rare. Vomiting in "ictus emeticus" develops after the patient has lost consciousness. Patients do not recall vomiting, unless they see the vomitus when they awaken. Upset stomach and a need to urinate or defecate often precede or follow syncope. Sweating and pallor are common features of faints.

Demography may also be helpful. Seizures occur at any age, whereas TIAs are not very common in young individuals, especially in those who do not have prominent risk factors for vascular disease, such as hypertension, diabetes, smoking, cardiac disease, sickle cell disease, and the like. Syncope has little predilection for age. Syncope is more common in women. TIAs and strokes are somewhat more common in men, although after menopause, the frequencies are nearly equal in the two sexes. Seizures have no strong sex predilection.

Differential Diagnosis of Persistent Neurologic Deficits with Relatively Abrupt Onset Strokes are characterized by the abrupt or at least very acute onset of focal neurologic symptoms and signs that leave persistent neurologic deficits. Other disorders that have acute onsets and cause persistent focal signs should be considered in the differential diagnosis.

Brain tumors can cause an abrupt onset or worsening of symptoms. Hemorrhage into a tumor is one mechanism for abrupt change. When some tumors, such as meningiomas, which are outside the brain, reach a critical mass, they can cause abrupt displacement of brain tissue and sudden onset of symptoms. Nonketotic hyperglycemic stupor often is associated with focal neurologic signs, and there may be a focal region of brain edema on brain imaging tests (CT or magnetic resonance imaging [MRI]). Attacks of multiple sclerosis (MS) can begin abruptly. Most often, however, MS attacks develop during 5 to 21 days, a longer period than strokes. MS is most common in the second to fourth decades of life, whereas the frequency of stroke peaks later. A history of prior attacks is very important in diagnosis. Demyelinization (acute disseminated encephalomyelitis [ADEM]) can occur after various viral infections and can cause the abrupt onset of multifocal signs that develop over days. Viral infections, especially cytomegalovirus (CMV) and herpes zoster varicella (HZV) virus, can cause focal brain lesions associated with focal neurologic signs. Brain abscesses cause focal neurologic symptoms and signs, and the disorder can begin rather abruptly. Fever, headache, and seizures are common accompanying signs.

Epileptic seizures, especially repeated focal seizures, can be followed by postictal paralysis or loss of other functions.

Imaging and Laboratory Tests Whenever possible, every patient suspected of having a stroke or TIA should have a brain image performed. The presence of a brain infarct on CT or MRI scans, especially in an area suggested by the localization of the TIA or stroke—for example, in the left precentral gyrus or left internal capsule in a patient with transient right arm and leg weakness—identifies a vascular etiology. Many patients whose clinical history and neurologic examination suggest that an attack was transient have infarcts in brain areas appropriate to the neurologic symptoms. The finding of an appropriate vascular lesion that correlates with the symptoms is very helpful in diagnosis. For example, in a patient with intermittent symptoms referable to the right arm or leg or language, a severe stenosis of the left internal carotid or middle cerebral artery makes an ischemic etiology very highly probable. The corollary is that the absence of a suitable vascular lesion raises doubt about the diagnosis of TIA or stroke. The appearance of lesions on CT or MRI scans often identifies nonvascular etiologies such as tumors, abscesses, subdural hematomas, or demyelinating lesions. Ultrasound, both extracranial and transcranial, CT angiography (CTA), and magnetic resonance angiography (MRA), are all noninvasive tests that can safely and quickly identify vascular occlusive lesions within the large extracranial and intracranial arteries. Echocardiography and cardiac rhythm monitoring can be helpful diagnostically by showing a source of cardiac-origin emboli. Blood tests can identify abnormal coagulability that can represent the primary cause of strokes or can complicate other conditions.

The laboratory evaluation of stroke patients should be question-based, because tests are chosen depending on the questions asked. The choice of tests should be sequential, because the selection of the second test often depends on the results of the first investigation. For example, if initial brain imaging tests reveal a hemorrhage, then the tests chosen will be quite different than if the initial scans show a brain infarct.

Question 1. Is the Brain Lesion Due to Ischemia or Hemorrhage? Brain imaging such as CT and/or MRI can invariably answer this question. Intracerebral hemorrhages show nearly instantly after onset as focal, white, hyperdense lesions within the brain substance on CT scans. Intracerebral hemorrhages also can be defined on MRI, especially if susceptibility (T2 weighted) images are included. Gradient-echo images can also show the presence of old hemorrhages, because this technique is very sensitive to hemosiderin, which remains in old hemorrhages indefinitely. Small SAHs can be missed by either CT or MRI, and lumbar puncture may be needed to show bleeding into the CSF. MRI is more sensitive than CT for the early diagnosis of brain infarction. Fluid-attenuated inversion recovery (FLAIR) images and diffusion-weighted images (DWI-MRI) are especially useful in showing infarcts early after the onset of symptoms. In patients with brain ischemia who do not yet have brain infarction, both CT and MRI may be normal.

Question 2. What If the Lesion Is an ICH? The location and appearance of the lesion, as well as the demography and risk factors of the patient (race, blood pressure, presence of known bleeding disorder, use of drugs, etc.), help decide on the choice of studies. CT scans usually define the size, location, and drainage pattern of intracerebral hematomas. Mass effect caused by the intracerebral mass, shift of midline structures, herniations of brain contents from one compartment to another, and the presence of hydrocephalus also are seen readily on CT scans. The appearance of the lesion, especially whether there is an underlying vascular malformation or a brain tumor, is more readily seen on MRI scans compared to CT.

If the patient is severely hypertensive, and the hematoma is well circumscribed, homogeneous, and is in a typical location for hypertensive ICH (putamen/internal capsule, caudate nucleus, thalamus, pons, or cerebellum), then ordinarily no further diagnostic tests are necessary. The clinician can be confident that the patient has a hypertensive hemorrhage.

If the patient has had recent trauma, and the lesions have the location and appearance of contusions and traumatic hemorrhages (anterior and/or orbital frontal lobes and temporal lobes at the surface), then a traumatic lesion can be diagnosed with confidence. Screening of bleeding functions (platelet count, prothrombin time, activated partial thromboplastin time, etc.) should be ordered in every patient with an intracranial hemorrhage, especially if the cause is not immediately clear. A bleeding tendency can cause or contribute to bleeding initiated by other etiologies. The prescription of anticoagulants is the most common bleeding disorder leading to brain hemorrhages. These bleeds are most often lobar or cerebellar. Anticoagulant hemorrhages often develop slowly, and may gradually enlarge over hours or even a few days.

If the hemorrhage is lobar or atypical in appearance, then amyloid angiopathy, bleeding into a tumor, and vascular malformations are likely possibilities. Hemorrhages related to amyloid angiopathy are mostly lobar but occasionally cerebellar. They involve mostly the posterior portions of the brain—the parietal and occipital lobes. They are usually multiple. Gradient-echo MRI may show the presence of old, small hemorrhages. Patients with amyloid angiopathy are usually over 65 years old. If the patients is young (under 60), the hemorrhage is lobar, and the blood pressure is not sufficiently elevated to make a firm diagnosis of hypertensive lobar hemorrhage, then other bleeding lesions should be excluded by further tests. A repeat MRI after the blood has been reabsorbed (4 to 8 weeks) often will show residual vascular malformations and brain tumors if such are present. Vascular imaging using either CT angiography (CTA) or MR angiography (MRA) of the intracranial circulation are useful screening tests for vascular malformations and aneurysms. In some patients, especially when vascular malformations or aneurysms are suspected by the screening vascular examinations, contrast angiography by arterial catheterization is warranted. Patients with intracerebral hemorrhage after cocaine (but not amphetamine) ingestion have a relatively high incidence of aneurysms and vascular malformations. They require vascular imaging tests (CTA, MRA, and/or angiography).

Question 3. What If the Bleeding Is Subarachnoid (SAH)? The most important cause of subarachnoid hemorrhage is rupture of an aneurysm on the surface of the brain into the subarachnoid space. Sudden severe headache, loss of attention, vomiting, and alteration in the state of alertness (restless and agitated or sleepy) are the usual clinical findings. A CT scan will show large acute SAHs, but smaller or less acute (more than 2 days old) bleeds may not be visible on CT. If the diagnosis is uncertain, a lumbar puncture is mandatory. When SAH is discovered, vascular imaging (usually angiography) should be performed. In older patients who may not be good candidates for surgery, CTA or MRA could be used as screening vascular examinations.

In one type of relatively benign SAH, the blood is centered around the brainstem (so-called perimesencephalic hemorrhage). This type of hemorrhage is usually not related to an aneurysm.

In patients with aneurysmal SAH, the location of the blood and its extent can help localize the site of the bleeding, and this also is helpful in predicting the likelihood of cerebral vascular vasoconstriction ("vasospasm") as a complication of the SAH.

Other causes of SAH include head trauma, bleeding diatheses, amyloid angiopathy, drug use (especially cocaine and amphetamines), vascular malformations, and tumors near the surface of the brain. At times, the blood is derived from a spinal vascular malformation. As in cocaine-related ICH, SAH after cocaine ingestion warrants angiography, because the frequency of aneurysms is high.

Question 4. What If the Problem Is Brain Ischemia? If the brain imaging shows infarction or at least does not show hemorrhage, then the diagnosis of brain ischemia is highly likely. Brain ischemia is a cerebrovascular disease. Every effort should be made to define the causative cardiac-hematologic-cerebrovascular condition in each patient, because treatment depends on the causative vascular lesion. Brain imaging alone is not sufficient investigation for a patient with transient or persisting brain ischemia.

When a brain infarct is present on CT or MRI, the first step is to characterize the location and size of the infarct. In general, it is useful to divide infarcts into those that are:

1. Subcortical and small—potentially within the blood supply of a single penetrating artery. The most frequent locations of such small deep infarcts are the basal ganglia, internal capsule, thalamus, and pons.
2. Large subcortical infarcts, larger than could be readily explained by occlusion of a single penetrating artery
3. Cortical infarcts—Infarcts limited to the cerebral cortex.
4. Infarcts that are cortical and subcortical
5. Brainstem and cerebellar infarcts that do not fit into category 1.

If the patient has a small deep infarct (category 1), then the most common cause is lacunar infarction caused by degenerative changes in penetrating arteries. Most such patients have risk factors for penetrating artery disease (hypertension and/or diabetes, or polycythemia), and the clinical findings most often conform to one of the well-recognized lacunar syndromes—pure motor hemiparesis, pure sensory stroke, dysarthria clumsy hand, or ataxic hemiparesis. In patients suspected of having lacunar infarction who have all three congruent findings (i.e., typical risk factors, clinical neurologic findings, and brain imaging), other testing has a low yield. Many clinicians perform vascular imaging (CTA or MRA) at the same time as brain imaging (CT or MRI) to exclude occlusion of the parent feeding artery, a condition that can mimic lacunar infarction. Because intracranial large artery occlusive disease is quite common in blacks and persons of Asian descent, it is especially important to perform intracranial vascular imaging in these patients. An alternative diagnostic test to exclude intracranial occlusive disease is transcranial Doppler ultrasound (TCD), a technique that measures blood flow velocities in the large intracranial arteries using an ultrasound probe placed over the orbit, temporal bones, and foramen magnum.

The other categories of infarction most often are caused by brain embolism or ischemia related to occlusive disease of the large extracranial and intracranial cervicocranial arteries. Infarcts that are large and subcortical often are caused by occlusion of intracranial arteries. Usually, in these patients, the stroke is preceded by TIAs, the onset is not abrupt, and the course of neurologic symptoms and signs fluctuates or progresses. Both intracranial and extracranial vascular testing are important. Extracranial vascular testing can be performed using MRA, CTA, or duplex ultrasound. All are reliable and specific for detecting important severe occlusive lesions in the extracranial carotid and vertebral arteries. Newer ultrasound devices, such as color-flow Doppler imaging, improve the resolution and quantification of carotid and vertebral artery lesions.

Brain embolism is the most frequent cause of cortical and subcortical infarcts. Emboli can arise from the heart, aorta, and the proximal arteries in the neck and head. The recipient artery cannot know where the embolic material arose; it only shows that it is blocked by something. Embolism is especially likely when:

- The onset is sudden, and the neurologic deficit is maximal right from the beginning.
- The infarct is large, and the neurologic deficit is severe.
- A known cardiac or large-artery lesion is present.
- The infarct is or becomes hemorrhagic on CT or MRI.
- Multiple cortical or cortical/subcortical infarcts are present in different vascular territories.
- Clinical findings improve quickly (so-called "spectacular shrinking deficit").

A recent important advance in the detection of brain embolism is monitoring using TCD. Emboli that pass under ultrasound probes make a high-pitched chirp and are recorded as high-intensity transient signals (HITS). The location and pattern of these emboli can help define the presence of embolism and give clues to their source. TCD monitoring also can be helpful in assessing the effectiveness of treatment.

Cardiac evaluation is important in nearly all patients with brain ischemia. Cardiac and aortic emboli are very common. Many patients with cerebrovascular occlusive disease have concurrent coronary artery disease that is important to recognize. A thorough history, looking for evidence of symptoms of cardiac ischemia and arrhythmias, careful examination of the heart, and an electrocardiogram are important in every patient. Many will also need echocardiography. Transthoracic echocardiography (TTE) usually is performed first, but when the clinical picture suggests embolism, and the TTE and preliminary cardiac and vascular imaging tests do not clarify the cause of brain ischemia, a TEE is needed to examine the atria, atrial septal region, and the aorta.

The extracranial and intracranial arteries are also common sources of brain embolism. Both the extracranial and intracranial arteries should be studied. When the infarct and brain symptoms are within the anterior circulation (carotid artery supply), then the extracranial and intracranial carotid arteries and their middle and anterior cerebral artery branches should be the focus of the examinations. When the symptoms and signs and infarction is within the posterior circulation (vertebro-basilar system), then the extracranial and intracranial vertebral arteries, the basilar artery, and the posterior cerebral arteries should be the focus of the vascular investigations. There is no reason why patients with posterior circulation ischemia should be studied less adequately than anterior circulation disease patients.

The anterior circulation can be studied using duplex ultrasound of the neck and TCD of the intracranial arteries. The B-mode images of the carotid artery also give evidence of the degree of stenosis and irregularities or ulcerations within plaques. The morphology of carotid artery plaques is well shown by duplex ultrasonography. Alternatively, CTA or MRA of the neck and head arteries often is adequate. Angiography is used when the screening tests do not sufficiently define the vascular lesions and more characterization is needed, and when interventional treatment through an arterial catheter (angioplasty or intra-arterial thrombolysis) is considered. Within the posterior circulation, duplex and color-flow Doppler investigation of the origins of the vertebral arteries, and ultrasound of the subclavian arteries (especially when the radial pulse or blood pressure on one side is lower than the other) can suggest lesions of the proximal portion of the vertebral arteries. Atherosclerosis most often affects this region. The ultrasonographer can then insonate over the rest of the vertebral artery in the neck using a continuous-wave Doppler (C-W Doppler) to detect direction of flow within the artery (craniad as would be normal, or reversed, or to-and-fro flow suggesting proximal obstruction). CTA and MRA of the neck vertebral arteries also are helpful, but these tests often do not adequately show the origins of the vertebral arteries well. CTA or MRA of the intracranial vertebral and basilar arteries are important. Sometimes the films are cut too low so that the proximal portions of the arteries (just after they penetrate the dura to enter the head) are not shown. The clinician must be certain that the films are adequate to see all the intracranial vertebrobasilar arterial system.

Blood tests are necessary in every patient with brain ischemia. Every patient should have (a) complete blood count, including hemoglobin, HCT, WBC, and platelet count; (b) PTT and PT; (c) serum fibrinogen level; and (d) blood lipids, including total and HDL and LDL cholesterol and triglycerides. When hypercoagulability is suggested by the clinical findings or preliminary blood tests, then a coagulation battery should be performed. This should include measuring the levels of Factor VII and VIII, von Willebrand factor, antithrombin III, protein C, and protein S, and tests for activated protein C resistance and mutations in the prothrombin gene, and antiphospholipid antibodies (anticardiolipins and lupus anticoagulant). In patients suspected of having a hemoglobinopathy, a hemoglobin electrophoresis is warranted. In selected patients, a sedimentation rate, tests for Lyme disease, syphilis, and human immunodeficiency virus (HIV)

are warranted. Hyperviscosity and abnormalities of Ca^{++} metabolism can also contribute to or cause brain ischemia.

Question 5. Are Other Special Tests Useful in Patients with Brain Ischemia? Other tests can help further define and quantify ischemia and its cause, and thus help guide treatment and prognostication. The technology to image the brain and its circulation has advanced rapidly. Newer MRI techniques are very helpful, especially in the acute evaluation of patients with brain ischemia. Diffusion-weighted MRI (DWI) is a technique that is very sensitive for the presence of edema in the tissues. Acute infarcts and ischemic regions show very early on DWI scans before they are seen on CT or standard T2- weighted MRI scans. At the same time as DWI examinations, MRAs can be performed to show vascular occlusions. Perfusion-weighted MRI scans (PWI) can show regions of underperfused brain, which can then be directly compared to the brain already showing edema as detected by DWI. The brain that is underperfused but not infarcted (perfusion defect is greater than DWI defect) is at great risk of becoming infarcted if blood flow is not quickly restored to the ischemic region.

Single photon emission computed tomography (SPECT), and xenon-enhanced CT scans are other ways of imaging those regions of the brain that are underperfused. Positron emission tomography (PET) scans show the brain's metabolism functions for glucose and oxygen and also image blood flow, but this technique is expensive and not widely available, especially for study of acute patients.

Electroencephalograms (EEGs) are helpful in patients suspected of having seizures.

Genetic testing is useful in some patients suspected of having familial or genetically mediated disorders, such as mitochondrial disorders.

REFERENCES

Albers G, Caplan LR, Easton JD, et al. Transient ischemic attack–proposal for a new definition. *N Engl J Med* 2002;347:1713–16.

Caplan LR. *Stroke a Clinical Approach*, 3rd ed. Boston: Butterworth-Heinemann, 2000.

Caplan LR. *Posterior Circulation Disease. Clinical Findings, Diagnosis, and Management.* Boston: Blackwell Science 1996.

Caplan LR. Brain ischemia mimics; Clinical diagnosis of stroke subtypes, Laboratory evaluation of stroke patients. Up-to-date

Caplan LR. TIAs—We need to return to the question, what is wrong with Mr. Jones? *Neurology* 1988;38:791–93.

Caplan LR. Diagnosis and treatment of ischemic stroke. *JAMA* 1991;266:2413–18.

Caplan LR. Intracerebral hemorrhage. *Lancet* 1992;339:656–58.

Caplan LR, Gorelick PB, Hier DB. Race, sex, and occlusive vascular disease. *Stroke* 1986:

Fisher M, Prichard JW, Warach S. New magnetic resonance techniques for acute ischemic stroke. *JAMA* 1995;274:908–11.

Kase CS, Caplan LR. *Intracerebral Hemorrhage.* Boston: Butterworth-Heinemann, 1994.

CHAPTER 3

RECOVERY AND REHABILITATION

Karin Diserens, Gerhard Rothacher, and Julien Bogousslavsky

KEY POINT

- Neurorehabilitation is of profound value for the stroke patient and his social environment.

The recovery of neurologic functions often is observed after a stroke. Although many patients are left with profound disabilities, it is common for some patients to show variable functional improvement that can lead to near complete recovery. It is estimated that approximately 60% of stroke survivors are expected to recover independence and some 75% to walk independently.

Up until the last 10 years, the impact of rehabilitation on functional improvement was mainly empirical, depending greatly on individual experience and the medical system involved. Based on scientific proof, a rehabilitation program was considered a supporting measure but not a fundamental condition or even an important factor for recovery.

The degree and time course of recovery are not easy to predict at the onset of a stroke. The mechanisms have been difficult to identify in human beings. Nevertheless, new functional imaging techniques, initially used in experimental animal studies and then in humans, have contributed to understanding the mechanism of recovery and the role of neuronal plasticity.

This better understanding of cerebral functioning, however, demands a better understanding of rehabilitation techniques and their indications.

Increasingly, modern health care provision and its utilization require the consideration and evaluation of all economic aspects. Higher and ever-rising costs have prompted a search for greater efficiency in the delivery of stroke care. The appropriate management of stroke survivors in the rehabilitation setting has been identified as a major priority by the Agency for Health Care Policy and Research, which, in 1998, provided clinical practice guidelines of post-stroke rehabilitation.

The following chapter gives an overview of the development of the hypothesis of recovery in, the techniques used in, and measurement of stroke rehabilitation.

RECOVERY MECHANISM

Cortical Plasticity and Animal Experiences Since the pioneering work of, it is known that functional reorganization can take place in the adult nervous system. The classic experiments were first shown for input manipulation, in which the overuse or disuse of particular inputs led to an increase or decrease in the corresponding cortical representation areas. The pivotal question for restorative neurology was whether such plasticity also operates after cortical damage. Ablation of areas 1, 2, and 3 in the hand area of the primary somatosensory cortex of the monkey (SI) led to an immediate unresponsiveness on the hand representation in SII, the second somatosensory cortex, a functionally related but distinct cooperative area. Twenty-four hours later, the formerly unresponsive hand area was then occupied by a foot representation. It was observed that the cortical finger representations adjacent to partly damaged finger representations became enlarged in relation to rehabilitative treatment, whereas they remained unchanged in those monkeys not subjected to rehabilitative treatment.

Cortical Plasticity of the Immature Brain Many observations suggest that the immature human brain is characterized by *plasticity*—it is capable of major functional reorganization in response to external and internal stimuli. For example, children will recover language skills after sustaining a large insult or even hemispherectomy on the speech-dominant side if the damage occurs before age 7 or 8. Similarly, if a child with strabismus is forced to use the squinting eye because of patching of the good eye before about age 7, permanent visual loss in the squinting eye (amblyopia) can be prevented.

The sensorimotor system also demonstrates plasticity. Children with large unilateral brain lesions can learn to reach out and grasp an object and can walk, although with a limp. Movements of the paretic hand in these children are often accompanied by "mirror" movements on the opposite side. Such parallel movements are much more prominent when brain injury occurs before 1 year of age. These observations suggest that motor function might be represented in the hemisphere ipsilateral to the weak hand if injury is incurred early in life.

Functional magnetic resonance imaging (fMRI) was used to map the hand sensorimotor area of hemiparetic adolescents and young adults who had suffered unilateral brain damage in the perinatal period. Unlike normal subjects, who exhibit cortical activation primarily contralateral to voluntary finger movements, the hemiparetic patients' intact hemispheres were equally activated by contralateral and ipsilateral finger movements. Findings in 1993 are consistent with previous clinical observations and animal experiments, which suggest that the immature brain is able to reorganize in response to focal injury.

Reorganization of the Adult Brain and Functional Imaging

Position Emission Tomography Positron emission tomography (PET) allows the measurement of regional cerebral bloodflow (RCBF) changes elicited by the stimulation and activation of neurologic or behavioral functions. The focal changes reflect the distribution of cerebral structures associated with the activity under study. It is, therefore, possible to identify areas of the brain that are activated during the performance of a motor task. A study was made of the pattern of cerebral blood flow elicited during movement of the previously paralysed, recovered finger to the pattern of RCBF recorded during rest and the RCBF changes observed when the finger of the controlateral normal hand is moved. The results suggest that ipsilateral motor pathways may play a role in the recovery of motor functions after ischemic stroke.

In 1993, PET was used to study organizational changes in the functional anatomy of the brain in 10 patients following recovery from striatocapsular motor strokes. Comparisons of regional cerebral blood flow maps at rest between the patients and 10 normal subjects revealed significantly lower RCBF in the basal ganglia, thalamus, sensorimotor, insular, and dorsolateral prefrontal cortices; in the brainstem; and in the ipsilateral cerebellum in patients controlateral to the side of the recovered hand. These deficits reflect the distribution of dysfunction caused by the ischemic lesion. RCBF was significantly increased in the contralateral posterior cingulated and premotor cortices and in the caudate nucleus ipsilateral to the recovered hand. During the performance of a motor task using the recovered hand, patients activated the controalateral cortical motor areas and ipsilateral cerebellum to the same extent as did normal subjects. However, activation was greater than in normal subjects in both insulae; in the inferior parietal (area 40), prefrontal, and anterior cingulated cortices; in the ipsilateral premotor cortex and basal ganglia; and in the contralateral cerebellum. The pattern of cortical activation also was abnormal when the unaffected hand, contralateral to the hemiplegia, performed the task. In 1993, it was showed that bilateral activation of motor pathways and the recruitment of additional sensorimotor areas and of other specific cortical areas is associated with recovery from motor stroke due to striatocapsular infarction. Activation of anterior and posterior cingulated and prefrontal cortices suggests that selective attentional and intentional mechanisms may be important in the recovery process. These findings suggest that considerable scope exists for functional plasticity in the adult human cerebral cortex.

Functional Magnetic Resonance Imaging During 1992–94, functional magnetic resonance imaging (fMRI) techniques were developed to detect functional changes in the brain. The most widely used of these fMRI techniques is based on detecting local changes in blood desoxyhemoglobin concentration in active regions of the brain.

In 1993, this fMRI technique was employed to create functional maps of the hand sensorimotor areas of adolescents and young adults who were hemiparetic since birth. The active brain regions were displayed and characterized using integrated three-dimensional models of the brain structure and function of each subject. They compared the fMRI-derived cortical maps of the intact hemispheres of hemiparetic patients with similar maps of dominant (left) hemispheres of right-handed controls. They also produced fMRI-derived cortical maps of the motor areas of the damaged hemispheres of hemiparetic subjects. They found that the sensorimotor area in the intact hemispheres of the hemiparetic patients was substantially activated by ipsilateral (paretic) finger movement, suggesting reorganization of sensorimotor cortex in the human brain after neonatal brain injury. Another case is described in 1997, reporting the combined evaluation including electrophysiology and fMRI of cortical and cerebral reorganization.

Plasticity and Transcranial Magnetic Stimulation In 1998, transcranial magnetic stimulation (TMS) was used to investigate the properties of the corticomotor pathway and to map the primary motor cortex projection to hand and forearm muscles during a sustained isometric contraction in a group of subjects with writers' cramp of varying duration. Corticomotor threshold, motor evoked potential (MEP) amplitude and latency, and silent-period duration were normal on both sides in all subjects. The maps of the corticomotor projection were displaced relative to normal in all subjects and, in some cases, were distorted in shape, with extensions of the lateral borders and the emergence of almost discrete secondary motor areas. The degree of map distortion and displacement was greatest in subjects with long-standing writer's cramp (greater than 5 years), and was bilateral in some cases. The injection of botulinum toxin into affected muscles demonstrated that the alterations in map topography were not fixed and could be temporarily reversed during the period when the clinical effects of the injection were greatest, with the maps returning to their original positions as the effects of the injection wore off. It was concluded from this study that slowly evolving reorganizational changes occur in the primary motor

cortex in writer's cramp, and that these changes may be secondary to altered afferent inputs from both clinically affected and unaffected muscles.

In the human, changes in the MEP have been reported following stimulation of muscle afferents or nerves. Changes in MEP or map parameters also have been demonstrated in response to a wide range of sensorimotor effects, including voluntary contraction, acquisition of motor skills, in Braille readers, and following limb amputation.

These patterns suggest a degree of reorganization within the motor that may develop initially in a single or a few muscles, but that eventually may lead to a more general rearrangement of the motor output to multiple muscles in a manner that preserves the overall motor sequence of the classic homunculus.

Synaptic Plasticity Dynamic changes in the structural characteristics of the postsynaptic membrane and, in particular, of dendritic spines have been a topic of great interest during the last decade. Such changes are of particular interest because these tiny protrusions are the normal site of excitatory synaptic transmission in many regions of the brain, including the hippopcampus. Furthermore, changes in efficacy at excitatory synapses are thought to underlie many forms of adaptive behavior, including learning and memory.

During the last few years, several studies using fluorescent imaging techniques as well as electron microscopy (EM) indicate that dendritic spines can change their morphology and ultrastructure more rapidly than previously envisioned. Furthermore, electrophsiologic and immunohistochemical data suggest that glutamate receptors may be subject to rapid exo- and/or endocytosis, thus demonstrating that the biochemical composition of the postsynaptic membrane can be modified rapidly.

These findings were reviewed in 2000 and put into the context of synaptic plasticity of filopodial protrusions, developing a scenario of successive events that may underlie the major forms of long-term potentiation (LTP) and long-term depression (LTD) (Figure 3.1).

The Role of Reafferent Feedback It appears in Figure 3.2 that most patients

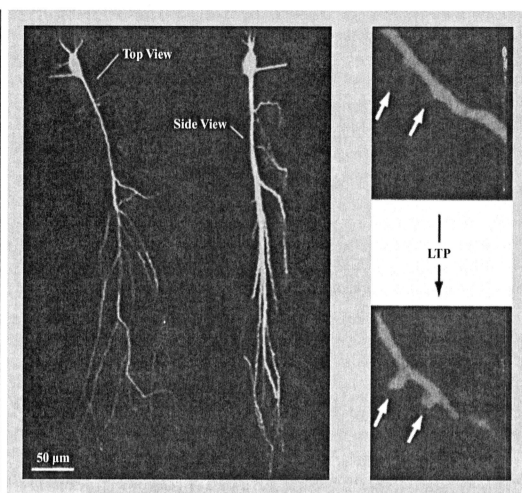

FIGURE 3.1 Structural changes of synapses. Proposed sequence of mechanisms involved in expression of LTP. Within 10 minutes of LTP induction, activation of Ca2+-dependent signal-transduction pathways results in phosphorylation of AMPA receptors and an increase in their single-channel conductance. In addition, the size of the spine apparatus increases, and AMPA receptors are delivered to the postsynaptic membrane by exocytosis of coated vesicles. This membrane insertion also leads to an increase in the size of the postsynaptic density (PSD) and, eventually, to the production of perforated synapses within the first 30 minutes. At 1 hour, through an unknown mechanism, some synapses use the expanded membrane area to generate multi-spine synapses (in which two or more spines contact the same presynatic bouton). Concomitant retrograde communication, possibly through cell-adhesion molecules, would trigger appropriate presynaptic structural changes, eventually increasing the total number of synapses.

recover well and early. The absence of any residual motor function seems to be a decisive, distinctive feature of severely affected patients who did not recover at all, when compared with a group of similarly affected patients who did recover completely. Evidence from combined clinical and electrophysiologic studies suggests that, in addition to the motor score, the presence of somatosensory evoked potentials (SSEPs) indicates good recovery. Furthermore, illusory arm movements also have been reported to activate beyond motor areas in the somotosensory cortex. It may therefore be assumed that the absence of residual function over a critical time span prevents functional

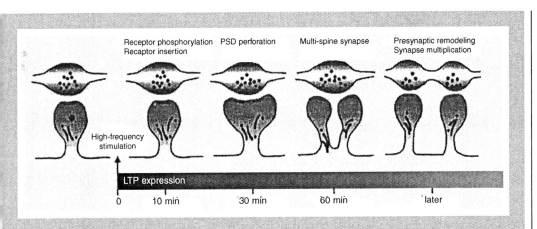

Receptor phosphorylation   PSD perforation   Multi-spine synapse   Presynaptic remodeling
Recaptor insertion   Synapse multiplication

High-frequency
stimulation

LTP expression

0   10 min   30 min   60 min   later

FIGURE 3.2 Intensive stimulation and structural changes of synapses. Analysis of post-stroke recovery shows three different groups irrespective of cortical and subcortical lesion location. Less severely affected patients with initial motor scores greater than 16 showed negligible recovery (n = 19) or recovered well in a longer time course (n = 16).

restitution. Conversely, animal experiments show an enlargement of the somatosensory representations during skill recovery after focal lesions of the primary somatosensory cortex. Further, deafferented monkeys who were not using the affected limb many weeks after injury failed to recover.

Although the lack of adequate afferent information may inhibit motor learning, discomfort and frustration may lead to overuse of the intact and non-use of the affected arm, the problem of *learned non-use*. Both improving afferent information and forcing the affected limb to be functionally active are basics for various therapeutic concepts. Thus, good evidence supports the view that reafferent somatosensory information from the partly compromized limb is critically required to tune the remaining network to function, as may be evident from scanning passive movements. These data are corroborated further by the observation that a posterior shift of the sensorimotor area occurs in patients with sensorimotor strokes (Figure 3.3).

Another modality that seems to play an important role in postischemic recovery is the visual system. Monkeys with focal ischemic lesions in the motor cortex visually inspect their hand when retrieving objects with the affected hand. In humans, it was observed that patients who had recovered from ischemic stroke differed significantly from healthy controls by the recruitment of a predominantly contralesional network, involving visual cortical areas and the prefrontal cortex, thalamus, hippocampus, and cerebellum during the blindfolded performance of sequential finger movements. Greater expression of this cortical–subcortical network correlated with a more severe sensorimotor deficit in the acute stage after stroke, thus reflecting its role for post-stroke recovery. Thus, a visuomotor brain system appeared to compensate for a sensorimotor deficit in patients who had recovered from hemiparetic stroke. This observation corresponds to animal models of focal brain lesions and to the developing human visual and auditory systems, suggesting that postlesional reorganization involves a network usually not active in sensorimotor activity.

In addition, it was shown that the lesion-affected and the recovery-related network in stroke patients shared the same structures in the contralesional thalamus and was bilateral in visual association areas. Thus, these sharing structures accommodated simultaneously passive lesion effects and active recovery-related changes in locations remote from the site of the brain infarction. This observation corresponds to the original conception of diaschisis as a restorative mechanism in functional recovery. That is, recovery is mediated by areas that have regained activi-

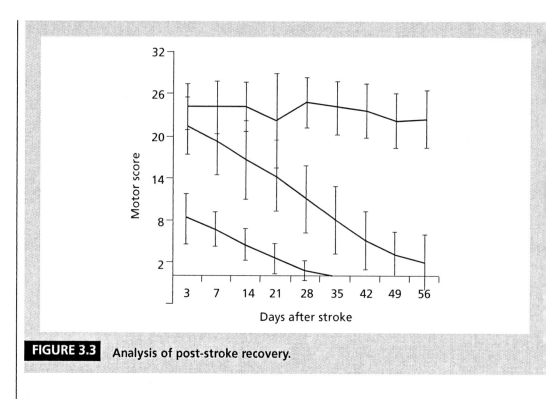

FIGURE 3.3 Analysis of post-stroke recovery.

ty after initial inhibition by a distant brain lesion. Thus, post-lesional reorganization appeared as a task-related rewiring of intrinsic cerebral networks. Whereas such a reorganization was shown to be effective in the perilesional vicinity, there seems also to be large-scale interregional reorganization. These affected regions did not show metabolic depressions in categorical comparisons with healthy subjects which, therefore, did not seem to be a prerequisite for the diaschisis. The type of activation-related interregional interactions suggests a task-related engagement of preexisting, hitherto latent pathways. Accordingly, when the functional changes evident from brain imaging correlate with neurologic deficits or with neurologic recovery, they may be referred to as instances of diaschisis and the regression of diaschisis. Similar conclusions also were proposed recently for psychologically impaired patients.

As evidenced by PET activation studies in patients recovered from hemiplegic stroke, such unused but functionally related pathways take on back-up or facilitatory functions. They may become engaged as alternative neural routes in patients with congenital or developmental brain diseases. From a phenomenological point of view, these cases represent temporary loss of function and its reappearance after a shorter or longer period of time. Disturbances of complete motor behavior, as occurs in neglect and limb kinetic apraxia, also tend to disappear with time. Nevertheless, ideomotor apraxia, visuomotor ataxia, and motor asphasia may be sufficiently stable in some patients or detectable by adequate neurpsychologic testing. As in the case of simple motor functions, the clinical presentation and resolution of these complex cerebral dysfunctions appear to be determined by the localization and size of the underlying brain lesion. In aphasia, however, the localization of the original lesion appears to vary more widely between subjects, reflecting the great variability of language localization. Also, some evidence suggests that large lesions in the frontal operculum induce a more severe aphasia.

An alternative hypothesis is that recovering patients select an alternative strategy to compensate for their neurologic deficit, as was shown in monkeys. A simple approach is that patients employ more extended finger movements for object exploration than they usually would. Thus, a spatially enhanced input is processed in a large portion of the sensorimotor cortex in these patients. Similarly, evidence suggests that patients with hemianopia can learn to exaggerate saccadic eye movements to compensate for their visual field defect. Likewise, hemiparetic patients may engage muscles for moving a paretic limb that are usually only used for auxillatory actions or reserved for high levels of exertion. This compensatory behavior is most prominent in patients with dystrophic muscle diseases (for example, while they are standing up or lifting a limb), but probably also holds for brain lesions. Finally, patients with Parkinson disease sometimes employ sensory cues to initiate locomotion. Clearly, these altered actions rely on abnormal sensorimotor or visuomotor information processing and are most likely to produce abnormal cortical activation patterns.

The Role of the Perilesional Area Plenty of evidence from experimental studies sugggests that the perilesional zone after focal ischemia is grossly abnormal. This does not refer to the concept of *penumbra*, which has been defined for tissue at risk during the first minutes and hours after the insult. Rather, the perilesional zone accommodates persistent and severe changes in tissue function in a surprisingly large area surrounding a lesion, as demonstrated experimentally. In the thrombosis model of the rat, small focal cortical lesions lead to changes that can be revealed by electrophysiologic, anatomic, and audioradiographic methods. Specifically, intracortical excitability is increased, intracortical inhibition decreased, and spontaneous activity and stimulus–response characteristics distinctly altered. These changes persist over many weeks. The implication of these prolonged changes for functional restoration and the cooperation of these perilesional areas with the remaining network are as yet unknown. Moreover, the perilesional area can be visualized microscipically using different staining methods in the histologic pictures, but they cannot be recognized properly even at high-field (7 Tesla) MRI, although its eletrophysiologic, audioradiographic, and metabolic patterns are clearly defined. Rather, neuroimaging in baboons and humans suggests that decreased labeling of

the GABA-B receptor indicated irreversibly damaged brain tissue.

For the clinician, this means that we do not see the remote changes. This is similar to the fact that we do not see relevant pathophysiology in basal ganglia, such as increased, spontaneous activity, abnormal synchronization, and the like, through imaging methods. Nevertheless, we must assume that this perilesional area is of considerable influence for the postischemic neurologic deficit and the pattern of functional restoration. The structural and the functional component of reafferent feedback emphasize that the old mechanistic view that the size of a destructed area is a major determinant for the resulting functional impairment is certainly too simplistic.

NEUROREHABILITATION OF STROKE

Definition According to the World Health Organization (WHO) definition, *rehabilitation* is a set of influences, procedures, and resources to be applied to the environment. Therefore, rehabilitation involves the prevention of disability and maintenance of social role, independency, and a meaningful life.

The processes of medical rehabilitation are well established in many countries throughout the world. A team approach is used regularly, involving physicians, rehabilitation nurses, physical and occupational therapists, speech-language-hearing pathologists, psychologists (including neuropsychologists), social workers, rehabilitation counselors, and recreation therapists. In addition, it is recognized widely now that the patient and family (significant others) are themselves integral members of the "rehabilitation team."

Each rehabilitation professional is licensed to practice his or her speciality. Guidelines and standards for structure, process, and outcome quality are elaborated worldwide but are not accredited in a homogenous way. These guidelines are important for quality control and for financing an expensive and long-term therapy, but consensus is difficult to achieve.

Only a few studies have been made of evidence-based care. The complexity of the rehabilitation approaches and the multivari-

KEY POINT

■ The benefits of rehabilitation outweigh the risk of harm to the patient.

able profile of the patients make a large randomized study difficult. Nevertheless, to control costs, attempts must be made to find good predictors for prognosis so that the appropriate orientation for the rehabilitation process can be established.

Following acute care, the program plan for rehabilitation must be elaborated. This includes a regular formalized functional reassessment using validated instruments and the establishment of the therapeutic goal of the interdisciplinary team and the patient.

Predictor Factors of Functional Outcome in Stroke Survivors Evidence from community-based studies provides valuable information on the expected clinical courses of stroke survivors as a group. This phenomenon has, perhaps, been best documented by The Framingham Heart Study. This research was carried out on stroke survivors from a community-based cohort (rather than an institution-specific study group, with the inherent biases this involves). It was, in addition, conducted with great methodologic rigor, including comparisons with age–sex matched control subjects from the same cohort who were free of stroke. The epidemiologic profile of 148 persons surviving stroke for at least 6 months is shown in Tables 3.1 through 3.4.

Table 3.1 displays the neurologic deficits manifested. Over half (52%) had no residual hemiparesis. Of those who did, equal numbers had left and right hemiparesis.

Dysarthria and dysphagia were associated more commonly with right hemiparesis. Otherwise, no striking constellations of residual neurologic deficits were observed and no significant difference was observed between men and women.

Stroke survivors had significantly greater cardiovascular comorbidity than the age–sex matched controls, with resultant implications for both survival and function (Table 3.2). They also had a significantly higher frequency of obesity, diabetes mellitus, and arthritis.

Table 3.3 displays the frequencies of nine different types of disability. Each disability was significantly more common in stroke survivors than in controls. Psychosocial disabilities (such as socialization and vocational function) were much more common than physical disabilities (such as problems with mobility or activities of daily living [ADLs]). The disability profile was not substantially affected after analyses designed to control for comorbidities.

Other recent community-based studies have added to this profile of functional outcomes in stroke survivors. In the Frenchay Health District Stroke Registry, 85% of enrolees were able to walk independently after 6 months, and 12% remained aphasic. Studies reviewed in the Agency for Health Care Policy and Research (AHCPR) guidelines found that two-thirds of survivors were independent in ADLs, results similar to those shown in Table 3.3. A 1984 Finnish study

TABLE 3.1 Neurological Deficits Manifested by 148 Survivors of Documented Completed Stroke—The Framingham Study (April 1972 through March 1975

Peripheral Motor Deficit	Defect Men	Women	Hemianopia Men	Women	Dysarthia Men	Women	Hemisensory Dysphasia Men	Women	All Patients Men #	%	Women #	%	Total #	%
None	4	1	3	2	1	2	7	6	31	47.0	46	56.1	77	82.0
Left hemiparesis	8	9	3	4	2	1	2	1	17	25.8	17	20.7	34	23.0
Right hemiparesis	5	5	2	2	8	7	5	5	16	24.2	17	20.7	33	22.3
Bilateral	2	2	1	2	1	1	1	0	2	3	2	2.4	4	2.7
Total	19	17	9	10	12	11	15	12	66	100	82	100	148	100

TABLE 3.2 Frequency of 14 Documented Comorbid Disease Processes in 148 Stroke Survivors and Stroke-Free Matched Controls—The Framingham Study (April 1972 through March 1975)

Type of Comorbid Disease	Stroke Survivors		Matched Controls		P
	#	%	#	%	
Hypertension	99	67	66	45	<0.001
Hypertensive cardiovascular disease	78	53	46	31	<0.001
Coronary heart disease	47	32	30	20	<0.05
Other heart disease	45	30	30	20	<0.05
Obesity	33	22	18	12	<0.05
Diabetes mellitus	32	22	15	10	<0.02
Arthritis	32	22	18	12	<0.05
Left ventricular hypertrophy by ECG	31	21	9	6	<0.001
Congestive heart failure	26	18	7	5	<0.001
Chronic lung disease	26	18	38	26	NS
Peripheral vascular disease	26	18	19	13	NS
Cancer	16	11	14	9	NS
Intermittent claudication	15	10	9	6	NS
Extremity amputation	3	2	0	0	NS
Total number of subjects	148	100	148	100	

ECG, electrocardiogram

TABLE 3.3 Frequency of Nine Types of Functional Deficit in 148 Stroke Survivors and 148 Stroke-Free Matched Controls—The Framingham Study (April 1972 through March 1975)

Type of Functional Deficit	Stroke Survivors		Matched Controls		P
	#	%	#	%	
Decreased vocational function	93	63	54	36	<0.001
Decreased socialization outside the home	87	59	42	28	<0.001
Limited in household tasks	83	56	30	20	<0.001
Decrease in interest and hobbies	70	47	30	20	<0.001
Decreased ability to use outside transportation	65	44	19	13	<0.001
Decreased socialization at home	64	43	41	28	<0.01
Dependent in ADL**	48	32	13	9	<0.001
Dependent in mobility	32	22	9	6	<0.001
Not living at home	22	15	3	2	<0.001
(nursing home or other institutionalized setting)	26	18	7	5	<0.001
Total number of subjects	148	100	148	100	

found depression in about 30% of stroke survivors at 12 months, and several studies have documented decreased quality of life after stroke. Gender seems to be a factor as well, with women more likely to be in institutions than men.

Rehabilitation Programs

Rehabilitation Reassessment and Outcome Measurements of Stroke Survivors Formalized functional assessment, using standardized instruments, is the means by which the levels of different types of disability are documented. This process of functional assessment is used to screen candidates for stroke rehabilitation, establish a baseline, document improvement, and establish final outcomes. In 1989, the WHO presented an important model, the International Classification of Functioning, Disability, and Health (ICIDH-1).

This model, with its negative connotations (disability and handicap), was modified in 2000 (ICIDH-2) and, in 2002, renamed the International Classification of Functioning (ICF) and modified to use more positive assessments of activities and participation as the measures of involvement in life situations.

These models have given therapists an organized structure for evaluation, goal-setting, and treatment (Table 3.4).

To establish the initial and final evaluation, measurement instruments must be applied. No single correct measurement of outcome for stroke patients exists. The choice of a particular scale depends on the type of underlying condition and the specific motive for obtaining the measure. Moreover, an outcome measure can be appropriated for a patient or a group of patients at one stage of their recovery, but not for another stage. In fact, given the natural history of stroke, change may continue over months, and the proportion of change may vary between the different levels of the ICF. The usual outcome scales are based on the WHO classifications, and they attempt to assess any permanent impairment, disability, limitation of activity, and restriction of participation, as well as the patient's conceptual context factors. However, the choice of outcome scales requires that they provide standardization among different examiners and institutions. Two elements are important for the selection of an outcome scale. First, the criteria in the scale must correspond with the user's purpose. The wrong choice can lead to erroneous results. Second, the scale must be reliable, valid, and appropriately responsive. Consequently, outcome measures must consider the timing of any assessment and the factors that can impact on the chosen outcomes. The method of statistical analysis also must suit the chosen outcomes.

The outcome variables that have been studied in stroke survivors include:

- Survival
- Location or living setting (e.g., within an institution or independent in the community)
- Walking (ambulation). Considered independently or as part of ADL, motor function, and balance

| | **TABLE 3.4** | Comparison of WHO ICIDH-1 and ICIDH-2 (ICF) |

WHO Model	Disease	Loss or Abnormality	Limitation of Activity	Social Consequence
ICIDH-1	Pathology	Impairment	Disability	Handicap
		Primary		
		Secondary		
ICIDH-2 (ICF)	Pathology	Impairment	Activities	Participation
		Primary		
		Secondary		

- ADLs. Basic self-care including feeding, toileting, dressing, transfers, mobility, bathing, and grooming
  - Independent ADLs (IADLs). More complex tasks needed for independent living, such as theuse of the telephone or public transportation
- Communication/speech and language function
- Psychosocial function, including cognitive performance and affect or mood
- Sexual function
- Community transition and social integration
- Return to work

The AHCPR guidelines contains a complete guide to standardized functional assessment instruments used in stroke rehabilitation. The more commonly used global instruments are reviewed here, and those limited to specific functional domains are included in the respective following subsections.

The *Rankin scale* was the first comprehensive functional assessment instrument published for use on stroke survivors. This scale provides an overall estimate of the level of functional dependence in a given stroke survivor.

The two most frequently used functional assessment instruments in studies of stroke outcome worldwide are the *Barthel index* and Functional Independence Measurement (FIM). Their properties are shown in Table 3.5. The Barthel index is limited to ADLs, but its great usefulness has made it a first choice for multiple investigators for 30 years. The FIM is newer but has grown rapidly in popularity. In addition to ADLs assessment, it contains items for communication and social cognition. It has been the vehicle for generating a large database on medical rehabilitation studies.

Patient progress should be monitored throughout rehabilitation using one of these standardized instruments, administered at

KEY POINT

- Treatment guidelines for stroke care should include medical, diagnostic, structural, and rehabilitative aspects that optimize the chances of stroke survival in the best conditions possible.

TABLE 3.5 Comparison of the Two Functional Assessment Instruments in Studies of Stroke

Instrument	Description	Validity, Rehabilitation and Sensitivity	Uses and Time to Administer	Strengths and Weaknesses
Barthel Index	Ordinal scale with total scope from 0 (totally dependent) to 20 (totally independent) (or, 0 to 100 by multiplying each item score by 5), 10 items: bowel, bladder feeding, grooming, dressing, transfer, toilet use, mobility, stairs, bathing.	Validity (i) Reliability (ii) Sensitivty (iii)	Uses Screening, formal assessment, monitoring, maintenance Time 5–10 minutes	Strengths Widely used in stroke disability Exellent reliability and validity Weaknesses "Ceiling" effect in detecting change at higher level functioning Only fair sensitivity to change
Functional Independence Measure (FIM)	16 items scored on a 7-point ordinal scale (1=complete independence, 7=total assistance). Total score ranges from 18 to 126. Subscores for motor function and cognition. Domains for self-care, sphincter control, mobility, locomotion, communication, and social cognition.	Validity(iv) Reliability (iv) Sensitivty (iv)	Uses Screening, formal assessment, monitoring, maintenance Time <40 minutes	Strengths Measures social cognition and cognition and functional communication as well as mobility and ADL. Use of a 7-point scale increases sensitivity v. other disability scales. Widely used in the U.S.+ other countries Weaknesses "Ceiling" and "floor" effects at the upper and lower ends of function.

ADL: activities of daily living
(i) Wade 1987; (ii) Wade 1988; (iii) Shah; (iv) Granger
From Gresham et al.

the time of entry into a rehabilitation program, at frequent intervals during rehabilitation, and during the first year after a patient returns to community living. The value of the information will be greatest if the instrument is administered in a consistent fashion by health professionals who are trained in its use. Results self-recorded by patients or their families are likely to differ considerably from those obtained by direct observation of the patient by professionals, and these must be cross-validated. The goals of evaluation are to document clinically meaningful progress and to identify areas in which the patient fails to progress. Lack of progress may indicate a need for changes in the treatment regimen or may suggest that further treatment is not warranted. Both FIM and the Barthel index have ceiling effects and, therefore, may not be sensitive enough to measure progress in patients with mild levels of disability.

The results of standardized functional assessment must be combined with certain other information to produce a complete evaluation of rehabilitation potential. Intrinsic items include age, sex, race, marital status, a detailed evaluation of neurologic deficits, ethiology of stroke, comorbid processes, educational level, vocational status, and financial, insurance, and entitlement status. Extrinsic factors also are important. These include the constellation of family or significant others; the physical environment of the home; and the physical environment, resources, attitudes, and services available in the patient's community.

As soon as the patient becomes medically stable after a stroke and the assessment is complete, a knowledgeable and experienced physician should review the profile of patient characteristics and decide whether and in what type of setting rehabilitation services or programs are indicated.

Selection of Setting for Rehabilitation Program One of the major contributions made by the AHCPR Clinical Practice Guideline on Stroke Rehabilitation was the formulation of a consensus-based decision tree for selecting the most appropriate rehabilitation setting for a stroke survivor (Figure 3.4. Alternatives range from no rehabilitation to single rehabilitation services to formal

rehabilitation programs of varying intensity. Settings can be free-standing rehabilitation hospitals or rehabilitation units in general hospitals, nursing homes, outpatient facilities, or programs delivered in patient's home. The goal is to match the stroke survivor's medical and functional status with the capabilities of available rehabilitation programs. It is imperative that the stroke survivor and her family or significant others participate in the decision about if and where stroke rehabilitation services are to be delivered.

Threshold criteria at the top of Figure 3.4 indicate patient characteristics that are essential preconditions for referral to any rehabilitation program. Reasonable medical stability, some significant functional disability, and the ability to learn and retain new ways of performing daily activities are primary among these. Medical conditions such as severe angina pectoris or inadequately diagnosed or treated infections militate against referral to rehabilitation until they are under control. Neurologic impairments that do not significantly affect the patient's ability to perform daily functions do not usually require rehabilitation therapies. Patients who are unable to participate in rehabilitation treatments because of cognitive deficits that result in the inability to concentrate or to learn adaptive strategies for performing tasks are unlikely to benefit from rehabilitation. At least some minimal level of physical endurance also is essential.

The choice of rehabilitation setting for a patient who meets threshold criteria depends most importantly on the level of assistance required to perform daily activities, the closeness of medical supervision required, the ability to tolerate intense and frequent therapies, and the availability of caregiver support. A patient who requires moderate or maximal assistance (50% or more of the efforts supplied by others) and can tolerate activities requiring intense physical and mental effort several hours a day has the potential to recover function more rapidly if referred to an intense ("acute") rehabilitation program in a hospital or nursing facility. Patients who are not able to tolerate intense treatments, even if they need moderate or maximal assistance, will be bet-

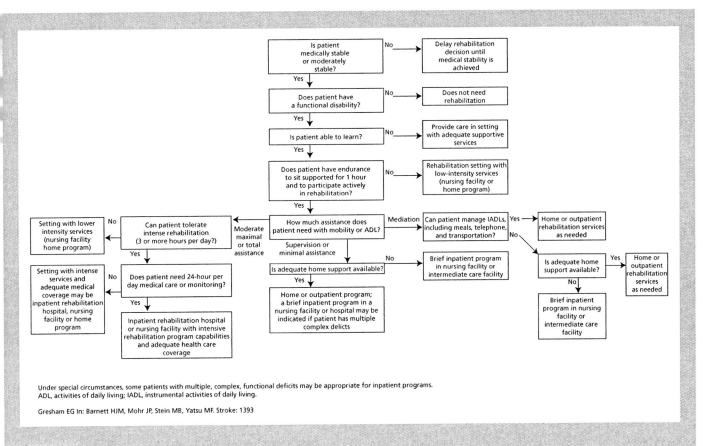

Under special circumstances, some patients with multiple, complex, functional deficits may be appropriate for inpatient programs.
ADL, activities of daily living; IADL, instrumental activities of daily living.

Gresham EG In: Barnett HJM, Mohr JP, Stein MB, Yatsu MF. Stroke: 1393

FIGURE 3.4 Propositions of selection of setting for rehabilitation program after hospitalization for acute stroke.

ter served in a lower-level program in a nursing facility or at home.

A greater flexibility of setting is possible for those patients with disabilities requiring lesser levels of assistance. In these situations, the availability of adequate support at home often determines whether an outpatient, home, or nursing-home program is best.

Process of Stroke Rehabilitation and Rehabilitation Techniques Rehabilitation is an integrated learning process aimed at assisting the patient to achieve the greatest possible return of functional independence after a stroke. A treatment plan individualized to each patient's needs aims to:

- Prevent recurrent strokes and complications of the stroke
- Reduce the effects of specific neurologic deficits
- Help the patient adapt to life in a community setting after discharge from a rehabil-

itation program and to maintain functional abilities over the long term.

An extensive literature discusses the process of rehabilitation. Current recommendations are largely consensus-based, although some conclusions can be drawn from research studies. In all cases, appropriate treatment plan documentation is required, periodic evaluation by the team or provider is mandatory, and a smooth transition to a permanent living setting (usually the home) must be effected when an inpatient rehabilitation program has been completed. Each of the following clinical or functional areas will be addressed during rehabilitation and, if indicated, specific treatment will be instituted.

The following aspects must be considered:

Prevention of Recurrence. The recurrence of stroke is a considerable (7% to 10%) risk during the first year. The choice of ther-

KEY POINT

- In respect to rehabilitation, the application of guidelines must be adapted to the individual capacity of the patient and the possibilities of the interdisciplinary team, including an expert with knowledge in stroke. These are the key features for effectiveness.

apy depends on the ethiology of the stroke. For patients with subarachnoid hemorrhage, surgical treatment is effective in selected cases to prevent rebleeding. Anticoagulation may be considered for a potentially cardiogenic source of embolism, as in patients with nonvalvular atrial fibrillation. Antiplatelet drugs, such as aspirin or clopidogrel, may reduce the risk of ischemic stroke in patients with TIA and minor strokes. The use of heparin during the acute phase for patients with progressive ischemic stroke or in patients with a more than 70% ipsilateral carotid stenosis prior to carotid endarterectomy often is performed. Continuous control and the start of long-term treatment of cardiovascular risk factors (e.g., hypertension, diabetes, or smoking) is mandatory.

Pulmonary embolism. Pulmonary embolism accounts for about 10% of deaths from stroke. Therefore, all stroke patients should be screened for deep venous thrombosis (DVT). Because immobilization increases the risk of DVT, prophylaxis with heparin should be implemented soon after admission and continued until the patient is sufficiently mobile. Pooled data has shown a 45% risk reduction using low-dose heparin and a 79% risk reduction using low-molecular-weight heparin (LMWH). The use of elastic stockings is also effective in preventing DVT.

Skin Protection. Measures to maintain skin integrity should be initiated during acute care and continued throughout rehabilitation. At highest risk for skin problems are patients who are comatose, incontinent, or with high spastic muscle tone. Systematic daily inspection of the skin, paying particular attention to areas over bony prominences, gentle routine skin cleansing, protection from exposure to moisture (e.g., urine), proper positioning, regular turning, and gentle transfer techniques help to prevent skin damage. A full discussion of this problem and recommendations for prevention and treatment is found in the AHCPR-sponsored guidelines.

Dysphagia. Dysphagia (impaired swallowing) frequently occurs in stroke patients and may lead to aspiration and pneumonia. Aspiration is silent in about 40% of patients who aspirate. The goals of dysphagia management are to prevent aspiration, dehydration, and malnutrition and to restore safe swallowing. In supratentorial lesions, spontaneous improvement is frequent and often fast, while brainstem lesions have a longer time frame and a worse prognosis.

Screening the patient's ability to swallow should be assessed in all patients soon after admission and before any oral intake of fluids or food. The screening procedure itself is done in an upright body position using small amounts of fluid and food, paying attention to dysfunction of the lips, mouth, tongue, palate, pharynx, larynx, or proxial esophagus. Video fluoroscopy and/or video endoscopy allow a more differentiated analysis of the swallowing problem and may help to guide treatment decisions. Compensatory treatments involve changes in posture and the position used for swallowing, learning swallowing manoeuvres, (e.g., Mendelson manoeuvre or supraglottic swallowing), changes in texture of food, (e.g.m thickening liquids, use of puréed food), bolus size, temperature, or route of administration (e.g., by syringe). Perenteral or tube feeding may be necessary, whereas long-term tube feeding preferably is achieved by gastrostomy. Evidence of the effectiveness of treatment is mainly supported by observational studies, because controlled trials are lacking.

Bladder Control. Problems with bladder control and incontinence are common after stroke but resolve spontaneously in the majority of patients. Long-lasting incontinence infers a poor long-term prognosis for functional recovery. (Its predictive significance [78%] is higher than other for factors, such as consciousness or daily activity autonomy [68%].) Urinary incontinence can result from bladder hypo- and hyperreflexia as well as from inattention, mental status changes, and immobility. Persistent incontinence should be evaluated to identify the most severely affected patients and treatable medical conditions, such as urinary tract infections. Indwelling catheter use should be limited to as short a time as possible because of the increasing risk of bacteriuria and urinary tract infections.

Urinary retention can be successfully managed through clean intermittent catherization. Persistent urinary incontinence after stroke should be evaluated to determine its ethiology. For further discussion of the management of urinary incontinence, see the AHCPR-sponsored guidelines, Urinary Incontinence in Adults (Urinary Incontinence Guidelines Panel, 1992).

Bowel Control. Alterations of bowel problems may be incontinence, diarrhoea, or constipation and impaction, the latter being far more common. An assessment of constipation includes careful documentation of past and present bowel habits, dietary and fluid intake, and activity.

Sensorimotor Rehabilitation Early mobilization of the patient helps to prevent DVT, skin breakdown, contracture formation, constipation, and pneumonia. It may vary from passive range-of-motion exercises to out-of-bed activities, depending on the degree of neurologic insult. It has positive psychological effects on both the patient and family, and contributes to reduce mortality and to improve functional outcomes.

Mobilization is recommended as soon as the patient's medical and neurologic condition permits and, if possible, 24 to 48 hours after admission. Mobilization must be delayed or done with caution in patients with coma, severe obtudation, progressing neurologic signs or symptoms, subarachnoidal or intracranial hemorrhage, severe orthostatic hypotension, and acute myocardial infarction.

The rate of mobilization depends on the general health condition of the patient, the underlying cause of stroke, physical endurance, postural stability, and the extent of orthostatic hypotension.

In 1999, the risk was shown for orthostatic reactions 2 to 3 weeks after stroke onset. Because, during the first week, a reactive increase of the systolic and diastolic blood pressure is observed, mobilization during this first week is recommended except in cases with severe vascular stenosis, very severe stroke, or severe cardiovascular diseases. Observation of symptoms during exercise, fatigability, blood pressure responses, heart rate and rhythm, and respiration compared to exercise ratio are important cues to evaluate endurance and thus decide on the rate and extent of mobilization.

TABLE 3.6	The NIH Stroke Scale: Relationship with Discharge Disposition
Admission NIH Stroke Scale Score	**Discharge Disposition**
0–8	Home with outpatient therapy (P = .001)
9–17	Inpatient rehabilitation (P = .004)
18+	Skilled nursing facility, subacute care, nursing home, or home custodial care (P = .001)

The beginning of mobilization requires a careful and thorough assessment of the patient's impairments and resources. Beginning with the neurologic and medical examination and basic functional observations and testing, the assessment will gradually extend to a systematic evaluation of motor function, cognitive function, emotional state, communication abilities, and ADLs, and an evaluation of the patient's premorbid condition and his potential family and caregiver support. Discharge planning should begin early. The National Institute of Health Stroke Scale (NIHSS), which measures the severity of stroke, may be used to guide the selection of an appropriate discharge setting during the acute care phase of management (Table 3.6).

The following sequence of mobilization may start at any point depending on the patient's condition:

- Frequent position changes in bed and daily passive and active range-of-motion exercises of the limbs, sitting up in bed, and then progressing to the edge of the bed.
- Sitting outside the bed in a chair or a wheelchair.
- Learning passive and active transfers from bed to chair, wheelchair to chair, toilet to wheelchair.
- Getting to a standing position; starting to walk, with an aid; walking on a treadmill, with an aid; walking alone.

- ADLs may start with grooming, eating, toileting, and dressing, and extend to more complex tasks.
- Mental activities, including communication, are as important as physical ones.

A painful shoulder occurred in 72% of the 219 hemiplegia patients after cerebrovascular accident in a study by Van Ouwenaller. This problem occured more often in patients having spasticity (85%) than in those with flaccidity (18%). The sympathic dystrophy syndrome (past term for complex regional pain syndrome, CRPS I), the association of pain and of autonomic dysfunction (edema, dysfunction of skin flow, skin dystrophy, changes of skin temperature), was present in only 23% of all cases but was seen more often in spastic patients than in flaccid patients (27% compared with 7%). Central localization and processing play important roles in the occurrence of acute vegetative dysfunction. In association, sensitive or perceptual deficits may lead directly to unawareness of injuries to the extremity or of subluxation of the shoulder, resulting in peripheral nerve lesions that might initiate a self-perpetuating vicious cycle of pain, followed by the full picture of CRPS I (Figure 3.5).

These results underline the importance of intervention and correct mobilization as early as possible to prevent autonomic dysfunction.

During mobilization, falls are the most frequent cause of injury in patients hospitalized with strokes, and hip fracture is a common complication. Special attention must be given to patients with balance problems, sensorimotor paresis, confusion, visual

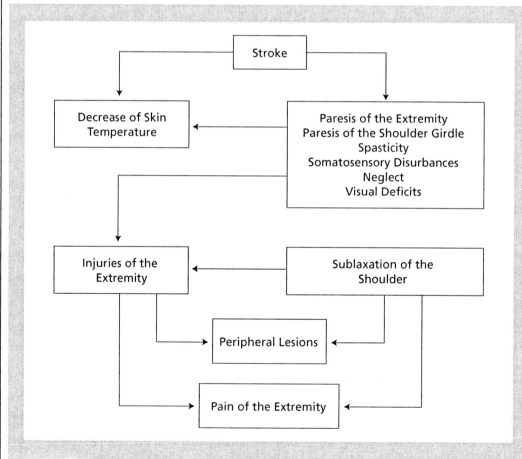

FIGURE 3.5 Hypothesis on the development of CRPS after stroke affecting upper extremity.

impairments, and communication problems. Patients with visual neglect or those who are slow in performing tasks have the highest risk of falling. Acute illness or drug effects may increase the risk of falls.

Perceptual Deficits: Unilateral Neglect Unilateral neglect or hemi-inattention is characterized by a disturbance in spatial perception affecting the contralateral side of the body. This deficit may occur in up to 50% of strokes affecting the right cerebral hemispheres and up to 25% of left hemispheric stroke. Neglect challenges independence in ADLs. The rehabilitation is an interdisciplinary approach. Clinical improvements can be achieved either by specific activation of the right hemisphere, as by transcutaneous electrical stimulation, or by compensatory strategies.

In a 1995 investigation of 14 patients with right hemisphere lesion, the effects of transcutaneous electrical stimulation on left visuo-spatial hemineglect were assessed through the performance of a visuo-motor exploratory task (letter cancellation). In Experiment 1, left neck stimulation temporarily improved the deficit in 13 out of 14 patients (93%), whereas stimulation of the right neck had no positive effects, worsening exploratory performance in nine patients (64%). Experiment 2 showed that left-neck stimulation temporarily improved neglect also when head movements were prevented by a chin-rest. In Experiment 3, stimulation of both the left hand and left neck had comprarable positive effects on visuo-spatial hemineglect. These results are interpreted in terms of: (1) nonspecific activation of the right hemisphere, contralateral to the stimulation side; and (2) specific directional effects of left somatosensory stimulation on the ergocentric coordinates of extrapersonal space, which in neglect patients are distorted toward the side of the brain lesion.

Communication Approximately 40% of stroke survivors will present a speech or language disorder (Post-Stroke Rehabilitation Guideline Panel). The impact of alterations in speech and language function may be devastating to the patient, reducing employability and quality of life and predisposing the patient to social isolation if not cautiously treated. When fluency of speech is altered by dysarthria, 'word-finding' errors, or the presence of an expressive, receptive, or global aphasia, a speech and language pathologist should be consulted early to assist with diagnosis and treatment.

Neuropsychological Alterations: Affective Disorders and Cognitive Dysfunction The incidence of post-stroke depression (PSD) has been reported to be as great as 68%, with major depressions reported in as many as 27% of stroke survivors. The origins of PSD may be organic, situational secondary to neurologic dysfunction, or related to comorbid medical conditions or drug therapy. Its relation to the localization of the brain infarct is discussed with controversy in the literature. Frequently, major depression occurs in strokes involving the left anterior cerebral cortex and the basal ganglia, whereas minor depressions and apathy occur most commonly in right posterior cerebral infarcts. An assessment for PSD should include the use of standardized depression scales, behavioral observations, and interviews of both the patient and family or other significant persons. Antidepressant medications coupled with psychotherapy may be used in the treatment of major depression.

Cognitive dysfunctions affecting the patient's orientation, attention, memory, insight, judgment, and abstract reasoning skills also may increase the length of stay during both acute care and inpatient rehabilitation, thus contributing to limited improvement in functional outcomes. A cognitive evaluation performed by a neuropsychologist should guide an appropriate selection of discharge options after completion of acute care management. Compensatory techniques and cognitive retraining, which includes repetitive exercises, may be employed in the acute-care phase of stroke management and carried through to the rehabilitation setting of choice (Post-Stroke Rehabilitation Guideline Panel). The long-term effects of these therapies have not yet been established in the literature.

Because cognitive alterations (e.g., disorientation, memory deficits, or misjudgement) are of great significance for social and vocational reintegration, and may cause severe problems and frustration in patients and care-givers, counseling and the teaching of "survival" strategies are of major importance.

In addition to rehabilitation programs, pharmacologic strategies have been advocated to improve the functional outcome and enhance the results of the neurorehabilitation of persons with cerebral lesions, either vascular or traumatic. Dopaminergic and cholinergic pathways have been believed to play a significant role in arousal. In 2005, an investigation followed 10 patients using a cholinergic agent (donepezil) therapy to treat chronic cognitive impairment due to traumatic brain injury. In a randomized, placebo-controlled trial Scheidtmann et al. showed improvement of motor recovery in 53 patients given 100 mg L-dopa prior to physiotherapy. Eight patients showed signif-

SUMMARY OF RECOMMENDATIONS

Rehabilitation following acute stroke:

Grade

- Acute inpatient care for patients with major stroke should be organized as a multidisciplinary stroke services based in designated units.

  A

- Rehabilitation should be started as soon as the patient's condition permits.

  B

- Rehabilitation aims, with short- and long-term rehabilitation objectives, should be established and agreed to by all parties including the patient and caregivers.

  C

Information provision:

- An identified member of the team should be responsible for providing information about the nature of the stroke, stroke management, rehabilitation, and expectations of outcome to the patient and caregiver, with full discussion of their roles in the rehabilitation process.

  A

- All information given to patients and caregivers should be documented to preclude passing conflicting information from different team members.

  A

- Information should be presented both verbally and in written form to the patient and family or caregivers.

  B

Continuing assessment and review:

- Assessment should be ongoing, taking into account the patient's changing needs and environment.

  C

- Post-discharge review should be arranged for 2 to 3 months after discharge. The date and location of such a review should be agreed to and documented prior to discharge.

  C

The role of the multidisciplinary team:

- Targets should be set for referral and assessment for each profession within the multidisciplinary team.

  C

- Hospital-based rehabilitation should be carried out by a specialist multidisciplinary team, coordinated by a consultant with a specific interest in stroke.

  B

- Stroke services should ensure an adequate level of nursing staff with appropriate specialist training.

  C

- Nurses should expand the realm of care to include family and caregivers of stroke patients, to ensure that they receive information in an easily understood format.

  C

- Physiotherapy should aim to promote recovery of motor control, independence in functional tasks, optimization of sensory stimulation, and prevention of secondary complications, such as soft-tissue shortening and chest infections.

  C

- The board role of occupational therapy in the rehabilitation of stroke patients should be recognized. Early referral for assessment is appropriate.

  C

- All patients with a communication problem resulting from stroke should be referred for speech and language therapy assessment and treatment.

  A

- Intensive speech and language therapy should be initiated as soon as the patient's condition is stable, and it may be required over the long term.　　B

- Where intelligible speech is not a reasonable goal, the speech and language therapist should increase speech attempts and enable communication through means other than spoken language.　　B

Prevention and management of complications of acute stroke:　　Grade

- Each hospital should have a guideline for swallowing assessment.　　B

- Urinary catheters should be used with caution, and alternative methods for the management of continence explored.　　C

- All those involved in moving stroke patients should receive training in safely moving and handling of the upper limb.　　C

- Low-dose heparin may be used for thromboprophylaxis in stroke patients considered at risk for DVT and PTE.　　B

- External compression stockings should be used where heparin is contraindicated.　　B

- The benefits of treating established DVT and PTE with heparin and warafin should be considered against the risk of using these agents in both ischemic stroke and primary intracerebral hemorrhage.　　A

- Awareness of the possibility of depression should lead to prompt evaluation and treatment.　　B

Discharge planning:

- An explicit discharge policy should be in place for stroke patients, to identify future needs.　　C

The evidence to begin rehabilitation as early as possible has been demonstrated.

icant positive changes in tests assessing speed of processing, learning, and divided attention.

Integration of the Social and Professional Context Factors Stroke is a catastrophe for patient and family. The survivors are confronted with disability and often experience a dramatic change of living situation and living plans. Families must learn to adjust to the altered relationship and to giving support to the disabled family member. Providing support to the patient and his family during this critical time, giving them (repeatedly) information about the nature of the disease and the consequences are important. Setting up goals, outlining the steps to reach these goals, explaining the nature and expected time frame of treatments, and providing empathy and emotional support may help to maintain motivation and must be a goal of education. Effective discharge planning will contribute to better outcomes, improve efficiency, and save costs. The patient and family should be intimately involved in the evaluation of needs and potential living options after discharge.

An important goal of discharge planning is to determine the need and the best setting for rehabilitation to ensure continuity of services after discharge. Figure 3.4 lists options for rehabilitation program settings after hospitalization for acute stroke.

Organization of Interdisciplinary Units (Stroke Unit) Epidemiologic studies showed the benefit of beginning neurorehabilitation as early as possible. The meta-analyses confirmed the hypotheses that well-organized interdisciplinary units diminished global costs. These units optimize the pathway from the beginning of the acute phase to returning home or to an institution.

Priority Listing for Recommendations of Rehabilitation Programs The Scottish Guidelines and the National Clinical Guidelines give a priority listing for recommendations of rehabilitation programs. (The definitions of the types of evidence and the grading of recommendations used in this guideline originate from the U.S. Agency for Health Care Policy and Research, as per Table 3.7.)

Level	Type of Evidence
	TABLE 3.7 Definitions of Types of Evidence and Grading of Recommendations (From the U.S. Agency for Health Care Policy and Research)

Level	Type of Evidence
Ia	Evidence obtained from meta-analysis of randomized controlled trials.
Ib	Evidence obtained from at least one randomized controlled trial.
IIa	Evidence obtained from at least one well-designed controlled study without randomization.
IIb	Evidence obtained from at least one well-designed quasi-experimental study.
III	Evidence obtained from well-designed nonexperimental descriptive studies, such as comparative studies, correlation studies, and case studies.
IV	Evidence obtained from expert committee reports or opinions and/or clinical experiences of respected authorities.
Grade	**Recommendation**
A	Required. At least one randomized controlled trial as part of the body of literature of overall good quality and consistency addressing specific recommendation. (Evidence levels Ia, Ib)
B	Required. Availability of well-conducted clinical studies, but no randomized clinical trials on the topic of recommendation. (Evidence levels IIa, IIb, III)
C	Required. Evidence obtained from expert committee reports or opinions and/or clinical experiences of respected authorities. (Evidence level IV)

Indicates absence of directly applicable clinical studies of good quality.

REFERENCES

Alexander MP, Naeser MA, Palumbo C. Broca's area aphasias: aphasia after lesions including the frontal operculum. *Neurology* 1990;40(2):353–62.

Anderson C, Mhurchu CN, Rubenach S, et al. Home or hospital for stroke rehabilitation? Results of a randomized controlled trial.II: cost minimization analysis at 6 months. *Stroke* 2000;31(5):1032–37.

Braddom RL. *Physical Medicine and Rehabilitation*. Philadelphia: WB Saunders, 1996.

Brandstater ME, Roth EJ, Siebens HC. Venous thromboembolism in stroke: literature review and implications for clinical practice. *Arch Phys Med Rehabil* 1992;73(Suppl):379–89.

Byrnes ML, Thickbroom GW, Wilson SA, et al. The corticomotor representation of upper limb muscles in writer's cramp and changes following botulinum toxin injection. *Brain* 1998;121:977–88.

Cao Y, Twole VL, Levin DN, Balter JM. Functional mapping of human motor cortical activbation with conventional MR imaging at 1.5T. *J Magn Reson Med* 1993;3(6):869–75.

Chollet F, DiPiero V, Wise RJ, et al. The functional anatomy of motor recovery after stroke in humans: a study with positron emission tomography. *Ann Neurol* 1991;29(1):63–71.

Cochrane Review. Stroke Unit Trialists' Collaboration. Organized inpatient (stroke unit) care for Stroke. Oxford: The Cochrane Library, Update Software, 2002.

Cochrane Review. Early Supported Discharge Trialists. Services for reducing duration of hospital care for acute stroke patients. Oxford : The Cochrane Library, Update Software, 2003.

De Lisa JA, Gans BM. *Rehabilitation Medicine: Principles and Practice*, 2nd ed. Philadelphia: JB Lippincott, 1993.

Diserens K, Rothacher G. Is early rehabilitation useful? In: *Recovery after Stroke*. Bogousslavsky J, Barnes M, Dobkin B, eds. Cambridge University Press, 2005.

Freund H-G. The Appraxis. In: *Diseases of the Nervous System*. Asbury AK, McKhann GM, McDonald WI, eds. Philadelphia: Saunders, 1994;751–67.

Gresham GE, Phillips TF, Wolf PA, et al. Epidemiologic profile of long-term stroke disability: the Framingham study. *Arch Phys Med Rehabil* 1979;60:487–91.

Gresham GE, Stason WB. Rehabilitation of stroke survivor:1389-1401. In: *Stroke Pathophysiology, Diagnosis, and Management*. 1998(3): Ed. Churchill.

Jenkins WM, Merzenich MM, Recanzone G , Neocortical representational dynamics in adult primates: Implications for neuropsychology. *Neuropsychologia* 1990;28(6):573–84.

Kelly-Hayes M, Robertson JT, Broderick JP, et al. The American Heart Association Stroke Outcome Classification. *Stroke* 1998;29:1274–80.

Khateb A, Amman J, Annoni JM, Diserens K. Cognition-enhancing effects of donepezil in traumatic brain injury. *Eur Neurol* 2005;54:39–45.

Luscher C, Nicoll RA, Molenka RC, Mueller D. *Nature Neuroscience* 2000;3(6):545–50.

Muller D. Ultrastructural plasticity of excitatory synapses. *Rev Neurosci* 1997;8:77–93.

National Clinical Guidelines. Rehabilitation following acquired brain injury. London, 2003.

Nirkko AC et al. Human cortical plasticity: functional recovery with mirror movements. *Neurology* 1997;48(4):1090–93.

Nudo RJ, Wise BM, SiFuentes F, Milliken GW. Neural substrates for the effects of rehabilitative training on motor recovery after ischemic infarct. *Science* 1996;272(5269):1791–94.

Nudo RJ, Frei KM, Delia SW. Role of sensory deficits in motor impairments after injury to primary motor cortex. *Neuropharmacology* 2000;39(5):733–42.

Panayiotou B, Reid J, Fotherby M, Crome P. Orthostatic haemodynamic responses in acute stroke. *Postgrad Med J* 1999;75:213–18.

Panel for the Prediction and Prevention of Pressure Ulcers in Adults 1992. Pressure ulcers in adults; prediction and prevention. Clinical practice guideline No.3 AHCPR publication no.92-0047. Rockville, MD: Agency for Health Care Policy and Research, 1992.

Paolucci S, Antonucci G, Grasso MG, et al. Early versus delayed inpatient stroke rehabilitation: A matched comparison conducted in Italy. *Arch Phys Med Rehabil* 2000;81:695–700.

Pascual-Leone A . Reorganization of cortical motor outputs in the acquisition of new motor skills. In: *Recent Advances in Clinical Neurophysiology*. Kimura J, Shibasaki H, eds. Amsterdam: Elsevier, 1996;304–8.

Roberts L, Counsell C. Assessment of clinical outcomes in acute stroke trials. *Stroke* 1998;29:986–991.

Scheidtmann K, Fries W, Muller F, et al. Effect of levodopa in combination with physiotherapy on functional motor recovery after stroke: a prospective, randomized, double-blind study. *Lancet* 2001;358(9284):787–90.

Scottish Intercollegiate Guidelines. Edinburgh: Scottish Intercollegiate Guidelines Network, 1998.

Seitz RJ, Azari NP, Knorr U, et al. The role of diaschisis in stroke recovery. *Stroke* 1999;30(9):1844–50.

Seitz RJ, Freund H-J, Binkofski F. Motor dysfunction and recovery. In: *Long-term Effects of Stroke*. Bogousslavsky J, ed. New York: Marcel Dekker, 2002; 122.

Stason WB. Can clinical practice guidelines increase the effectiveness and cost-effectiveness of post-stroke rehabilitation? *Top Stroke Rehabil* 1997;4(3):1–16.

Strüder HK, Kinscherf R, Diserens K, Weicker H. Physiologie und Pathophysiologie der Basalganglien; Einfluss auf die Motorik. *Deutsche Zeitschrift für Sportmedizin* 2001;52(12):350–60.

Stucki G, Cieza A, Ewert T, et al. Application of the International Classification of Functioning, Disability and Health (ICF) in clinical practice. *Disabil Rehabil* 2002;Mar 20;24(5):281–82.

Taub E, Miller NE, Novack TA, et al. Technique to improve chronic deficit after stroke. *Arch Phys Med Rehabil* 1993;74.

Taub E, Uswatte G, Pidikiti R. Constraint-induced movement therapy: a new family of techniques with broad application to physical rehabilitation—a clinical review. *J Rehabil Res Dev* 1999;36(3):237–51.

Vallar G, Rusconi ML, Barozzi S, et al. Improvement of left visio-spatial hemineglect by left-sided transcutaneous electrical stimulation. *Neuropsychologia* 1995;33(1):73–82.

Van Ouwenaller C, Laplace PM, Chantraine A. Painful shoulder in hemiplegia. *Arch Phys Med Rehabil* 1986;67(1):23–36.

Wade DT, Hewer RL. Outlook after an acute stroke: urinary incontinence and loss of consciousness compared in 532 patients. *Q J Med* 1985;56(221):601–8.

Wade DT, Hewer RL. Functional abilities after stroke: measurement, natural history and prognosis. *J Neurosur Psychiatry* 1987;50:177.

Wasner G, Schattschneider J, Binder A, Baron R. Complex regional pain syndrome—diagnostic, mechanisms, CNS involvement and therapy. *Spinal Cord* 2003;41:61–75.

Weiller C, Ramsay SC, Wise RJ, et al. Individual patterns of functional reorganization in human cerebral cortex after capsular infarction. *Ann Neurol* 1993;33(2):181–89.

Wojner AW. Optimizing ischemic stroke outcomes: an interdisciplinary approach to post-stroke rehabilitation in acute care. *Crit Care Nurs Quart* 1996;19(2):47–61.

Young FB, Weir CJ, Lees KR, for GAIN International Trial Steering Committee and Investigators. Comparison of the National Institutes of Health Stroke Scale with disability outcome measures in acute stroke trials. *Stroke* 2005 Oct;36(10):2187–92.

CHAPTER 4

STROKE IN DEVELOPING COUNTRIES

Luis César Rodríguez Salinas and Marco Tulio Medina

According to the World Health Organization (WHO), stroke is the second most frequent cause of mortality after ischemic heart disease, and the first cause of disability in adults worldwide. Globally, epilepsy (92.5%) and cerebrovascular diseases (84%) top the list of neurologic diseases most frequently seen by specialists. Stroke outweighs all other neurologic disorders combined as a cause of mortality, with an estimated 5.5 million subjects dying every year. Most of these epidemiologic data have been based on studies done in industrialized countries. However, published data during the last decade indicate that stroke is also a major public health problem in developing countries, where morbidity and mortality have reached an epidemic magnitude and represent an increasing challenge for the regional health systems. Today, two-thirds of stroke deaths occur in countries with low resources.

Recently published data from population-based studies showed a global crude prevalence rate ranging from 5 to 10 per 1,000 inhabitants. Projections for 2020 indicate a substantial increase in the annual number of victims, and the major percentage will occur in developing countries. Despite this, resources and services for dealing with these disorder are disproportionately scarce. Although neurologic services in Western countries vary from 1 to 5 neurologists per 100,000 inhabitants, neurology either does not exist or is only marginally present in Africa, South-East Asia, the Eastern Mediterranean, and the Western Pacific regions.

Hospital care, long-term care, complete or partial working incapacity, and lack of community support are enormous costs for patients, their families, communities, and the health care system. Hemorrhagic events are the most costly, and their prevalence in developing countries is higher than in developed countries.

ABOUT DEVELOPING COUNTRIES

Approximately 75% of the world's population lives in underdeveloped countries. Today, 1.3 million persons exist below the threshold of the absolute poverty level (income less than one daily dollar). Of these, almost 550 million live in Southern Asia, 215 million in Sub-Saharan Africa, and 150 million in Latin America, according to the United Nations. The life expectancy in these countries has increased from approximately 40 to 63 years over the last four decades. An inevitable increase will occur in the incidence of chronic diseases such as stroke. Africa is the poorest continent: 32 of the world's 48 less-advanced countries are African.

According to WHO estimates, three-fourths of the 51 million persons who died in 1993 were adult, and 39 million were living in developing countries. These nations are characterized by extremely fragile health systems and a shortage of adequately developed programs, especially for the prevention and control of chronic nontransmissible diseases such as stroke. Also, health budgets are low and opportunities for community interventions are small. Epidemiologic studies in these areas are usually flawed by incomplete case definitions and the lack of modern neuroimaging equipment. In 60.7% and 57.1% of low-income countries, no neurologic rehabilitation or neuroradiology services are available, respectively. Also, in 73.7% of countries in the Eastern Mediterranean and in 68.7% of countries in Africa, no stroke units are present, and these

- In 60.7% and 57.1% of low-income countries, no neurologic rehabilitation or neuroradiology services are available, respectively.

- The percentage of stroke recurrence seems to be particularly high in developing countries, reflecting poor compliance with treatment and inadequate control of risk factors.

- Tobacco constitutes an authentic plague, with more than 800 million of smokers worldwide.

- Trends in mortality from stroke do not necessarily reflect stroke occurrence in many countries.

- Latin American data reveal an annual incidence ranging from 35 to 183 in 100,000 and a crude prevalence between 1.7 and 7.5 per 1,000.

- Stroke prevalence in Latin America seems lower than that in developed countries, but this neurologic emergency is because of unknown protective ethnic factors or differences in dietary habits or lifestyles. Hospital-based stroke registries consistently report a high frequency of intracranial hemorrhages, which account for 26% to 46% of all strokes. High blood pressure, alcoholism, smoking, diabetes, and heart disease are the main risk factors for stroke in Latin America. Stroke in Latin America is related to some tropical diseases like Chagas disease, neurocysticercosis, snake bites, and malaria.

also are absent in 35.7% of countries in the Americas, 16.7% in Europe, 16.7% in South-East Asia, and 22.2% in the Western Pacific.

Those living in developing countries are unaware of the impact of stroke and usually do not seek prompt medical attention. Such delays result in more severe disease once the patient arrives at the hospital. The percentage of stroke recurrence seems to be particularly high, reflecting poor compliance with treatment and inadequate control of risk factors. Tobacco, which the WHO identifies as the most important reason of avoidable deaths, constitutes an authentic plague in developing countries. Of 1,10 billion smokers who exist in the world, 800 million live in these regions. Globally, smoking-related mortality is set to rise from 3 million annually (1995 estimate) to 10 million annually by 2030, with 70% of these deaths occurring in developing countries. These societies also face a growing epidemic of overweight and obesity, due to the frequent energetic imbalance between energy-dense food consumption and reduced daily physical expenditure. Differences in trends in risk factors, such as hypertension, diabetes, smoking, alcohol consumption, and diet, probably have the primary role in explaining the diverging trends in stroke mortality in different parts of the world. Added to these, a number of infectious and noninfectious conditions, highly prevalent in tropical countries, contribute to the high prevalence of stroke in these regions.

INTERNATIONAL TRENDS IN EPIDEMIOLOGY OF STROKE

The WHO data bank is an invaluable source of information for international comparison of trends. All those countries with low stroke mortality rates or those that show steep declines from their previously high stroke mortality rates during the last years are affluent, industrialized countries. Countries such as Japan and Finland, which had, respectively, the highest and the second highest rate of stroke mortality in the world during the early 1970s, are doing particularly well. Despite this, trends in mortality from stroke do not necessary reflect stroke occurrence in many countries. Data about stroke incidence are not always parallel with mortality. Although

declining trends have been observed in mortality, trends in incidence can be flat or even increase.

CURRENT SITUATION BY REGIONS

Latin America Stroke is a leading cause of mortality and disability in Latin America because of an increase in life expectancy and changes in the lifestyle of the population. In November 2004, the presidents of the Ibero-American Societies of Neurology assembled in Barcelona (Spain) to declare that stroke is a catastrophic disease in Iberoamerica. Few adequately designed epidemiologic studies have been reported in Latin-American communities. These studies reveal an annual incidence ranging from 35 to 183 (mean 96) per 100,000 inhabitants and a crude prevalence that ranges between 1.7 to 7.5 (mean 5.1) per 1,000 inhabitants (Table 4.1).

When these data is compared with developed countries statistics, stroke prevalance is lower. Nevertheless, this neurologic emergency is probably under-diagnosed in Latin America due to limitations in health and record systems. Some unknown protective ethnic factors or differences in dietary habits or lifestyles has been postulated as additional elements that could explain such difference. A need exists for more information about this point.

Hospital-based stroke registries consistently report a high frequency of intracranial hemorrhages, which account for 26% to 46% of all strokes. This is two to three times higher than that seen in people living in developed countries. Several factors may explain such differences, including a higher prevalence of uncontrolled arterial hypertension, poor dietary habits, widespread abuse of over-the-counter medications that predispose to bleeding, and alcohol abuse.

Profiles of stroke in the region also show some differences that are important for prevention and control strategies. According to published reports, 24% to 41% of strokes are atherothrombotic, 13% to 52% are embolic, and 13% to 42% are lacunar infarcts. High blood pressure, alcoholism, smoking, diabetes, and heart disease are the main risk factors for stroke in the region. Stroke mortality rates reported from countries like

TABLE 4.1 Stroke Epidemiological Community-based Studies Realized in Developing Countries During the Last 20 Years

Latin American*

Country	Date of Publication	Author	Incidence**	Prevalence***	Case-Fatality****
Bolivia	1997	Heckmann et al.	35		
Bolivia	2000	Nicoletti et al.		1.74	
Columbia	1997	Uribe et al.	89	5.6	
Colombia	2002	Pradilla et al.		4.7	
Colombia	1995	Pradilla et al.		6.5	
Chile	2005	Lavados et al.	140.1		23.3%
Ecuador	1985	Cruz et al.		3.6	
Ecuador	2004	Del Brutto et al.	64	6.38	
Honduras	2002	Medina et al.	65.6	5.7	
Honduras	2005	Thompson/Medina et al.		3.6	
Panama	1988	Gracia et al.		7.5	
Peru	1995	Jaillard et a.	183	6.2	
Caribbean*					
Barbados	2004	Corbin et al.	140		27.8%
Martinica	2001	Smadja et al.	164		19.3%
Africa*					
Sudafrica	2004	Connor et al.		2.43	
Tanzania	2000	Balker et al.	65		
Togo	2001	Balogou et al.		1.7	
Zimbabwe	1997	Matenga et al.	68		35.0%
Eastern Europe*					
Bulgaria	2002	Powles et al.	Males: 597 Females: 322		35.0%
Estonia	1996	Kory et al.	250		30.0%
Estonia	2004	Vibo	195		29.0%
Georgia	2004	Tsiskaridze et al.	165		47.8%
Lituania	1995	Rastenyte et al.	Males: 300 Females: 154		19.8% 21.3%
Polonia	1994	Czlonkowska et al.	127		
Polonia	1997	Ryglewicz et al.	Males: 123 Females: 64		38.0% 47.0%
Russia	1995	Feigin et al.	232		22.4%
Serbia	1991	Zikic et al.			42.2%
Ucrania	2001	Mihalka et al.	238–341		23.3%
Asia*					
China	2004	Shin et al.	219		
India	2001	Anand et al.		2.03	

* Community based studies
** Per 100,000 hab
*** Per 1000 hab
**** 30 day case fatality
Source: Who Data Base

- In the Caribbean, two community studies reveal an incidence of 140 to 164 per 100,000 and a fatality rate at 30 days of 23.5 %. The main risk factors for stroke are hypertension (69.1%) and diabetes (29.5%), higher than those reported in blacks from United States and United Kingdom.

- Hypertension is the major public health problem in most African countries, and noncompliance with hypertension medication increases the problem; unaffordable drug prices appear the major cause. Some studies have found high homocysteine levels among rural men and women in Africa, which could be explained in part by their marginal status with respect to folate and vitamin B$_{12}$ ingestion.

Argentina, Cuba, Ecuador, and México range from 23 to 72 per 100,000, with male predominance in most studies. Another particular characteristic of stroke in Latin American and the Caribbean is its association with tropical diseases and underecognized causes like Chagas disease, neurocysticercosis with vasculitis, snake bites, and malaria due to *Plasmodium falciparum* (Table 4.2).

Caribbean This region is composed primarily of a black population. The majority of published information is the result of reviews of hospital records, data that is not very useful to understanding the real epidemiologic situation of a disease. Two community studies reported reveal an incidence of 140 to 164 stroke cases per 100,000 population, and a fatality rate at 30 days of 23.5 % (see Table 4.1).

With regard to the types of stroke identified, in Martinique, Corbin et al. found cerebral infarction (IS) in 81.8%, intracerebral hemorrhage (ICH) in 11.9%, subarachnoid hemorrhage (SAH) in 2.0%, whereas 4.3% of strokes were unclassified (UC). Lacunar infarction was the predominant stroke subtype (50.7%). The main risk factors for stroke were hypertension (69.1%) and diabetes (29.5%). This population-based study showed a high stroke incidence and a high prevalence of hypertension and diabetes, compared with population from the United States and United Kingdom, probably related to inadequate control of these risk factors.

Africa The availability of basic and reliable data on cerebrovascular problems in Africans is limited, and this hinders the presentation of a comprehensive review of the subject. Nevertheless, evidence is strongly suggestive that the spectrum and pattern of cerebrovascular disorders in Africa is rapidly

TABLE 4.2   **Specific Disorders Causing Stroke in Developing Countries**

	Geographic	Distribution
Infectious Conditions		
Neurocysticercosis	Cerebral infarcts	Central and South America, Sub- Saharan Africa, Asia
Chagas' Disease	Cardioembolic infarcts	Central and South America.
Cerebral Malaria	Parenchymal hemorrhages cerebral infarcts	Central and South America, Asia, Africa
Tuberculosis	Cerebral infarcts	Worldwide
Viral Hemorrhagic Fevers	Parenchymal and hemorrhages	South America, Asia subarachnoid Africa
Leptospirosis	Parenchymal and subarachnoid hemorrhages	Asia, Central and South America
Infective Endocarditis	Cardioembolic infarcts parenchymal and subarachnoid hemorrhages	Worldwide
Noninfectious Conditions		
Sickle Cell Disease	Cerebral infarcts, parenchymal hemorrhages	Africa, Central and South America
Snakebites	Cerebral infarcts, parenchymal hemorrhages.	Worldwide
Cerebral Venous Thrombosis	Hemorrhagic cerebral infarcts	Asia, Central and South America

Modified and Reproduced with permission from: American Academy of Neurology, CONTINUUM. Stroke in the tropics.

becoming indistinguishable from that observed in developed countries. The classic risk factors appear to be on the rise, and smoking may attain levels equal to or exceeding those in many developed countries. Hypertension at frequencies exceeding 5% to 10% in most rural areas and 12% in most urban areas, together with complications such as stroke, heart failure, and renal failure, are leading causes of morbidity and mortality. Hypertension is the major public health problem in most African countries, and noncompliance with hypertension medication increases the problem. Unaffordable drug prices appear the major cause. It is thought that changes or modifications in lifestyle, risk-prone behavior, diet, cultural attitudes, and certain other consequences of rapid urbanization and demographic tendencies largely explain the observed trends. Some studies also found high homocysteine levels among rural men and women, which could be explained in part at least by their marginal status with respect to folate and vitamin B_{12} ingestion.

Although some epidemiologic studies of stroke and risk factors on the African continent have been published, a lack of well-designed community studies limits knowledge of the real epidemiologic profile of this disease in the region (see Table 4.1). Limited data are available on the stroke subtypes in Africa. In a hospital-based study from Tanzania, 60.1% of patients showed hemorrhage and 39.9% cerebral infarcts. Among the hemorrhagic group, 53.9% were men and 46.1%women, whereas 52.5% men and 47.5% women had infarction. Hypertension and diabetes mellitus were common risk factors in both subtypes of stroke. On the other hand, despite the high incidence of human immunodeficiency virus (HIV) in Sub-Saharan Africa, its relationship to stroke is similar to data from studies on young black African stroke patients who are HIV negative.

Eastern Europe Mortality from stroke has been declining over recent decades in most European countries, except in Eastern Europe. In the analysis based on the WHO Monitoring Trends and Determinants in Cardiovascular Disease (WHO MONICA) Project, undertaken in nine countries, an increase in stroke mortality was confirmed in Eastern Europe.

In the populations with a declining trend, about two-thirds of the change could be attributed to a decline in case fatality. In populations with increasing mortality, the rise was explained by an increase in case fatality. Whether this was due to changes in the management of stroke or changes in disease severity cannot be established on the basis of these results. According to epidemiologic studies, the case-fatality ratio in this region is between 19.8% and 47% (see Table 4.1).

Increased morbidity and mortality in Eastern Europe can be explained partially by higher rates in intracranial hemorrhages (18% versus less than 15% in Western Europe) due to the high prevalence of hypertension in this region. Other epidemiologic evidence favors poor nutrition, smoking, and alcoholism as the most important determinants of the differences in mortality rates between the regions. As an example, in Russia, cardiovascular diseases (heart disease and stroke) accounted for 65% of the cause of decline in life expectancy. Regional interventions are now directed to the early and opportune control of these risk factors

Asia and the Middle East The WHO database contains no records of community studies on stroke in the Middle East. In this region, some studies indicate that cardiovascular diseases remain a serious public health threat. In the Asia-Pacific region, countries such as Singapore have reported that cerebrovascular disease mortality has fallen over the last 25 years (from 99 per 100,000 in 1976 to 59 per 100,000 in 1994), in part related to the decline of stroke risk factors in the population.

Recent epidemiologic studies confirm that stroke is the most frequent cause of death in the People's Republic of China, with an incidence (219 in 100,000 people) more than fivefold that of myocardial infarction. Intracerebral hemorrhage causes about one-third of all strokes, nearly three times the frequency in North American stroke registries. A marked regional variation in stroke incidence exists, with a threefold higher stroke incidence in northern than in southern Chinese cities, suggesting important environmental or dietary influences. Some trials sug-

KEY POINTS

- Recent epidemiologic studies confirm that stroke is the most frequent cause of death in the People's Republic of China, with an incidence (219 in 100,000 people) more than fivefold that of myocardial infarction. Some trials suggest that tea drinking is independently associated with the prevalence of stroke and might play a role in the prevention of the disease.

- In India, a recent review of the information available showed stroke prevalence as estimated at 203 per 100,000 population.

- Cysticercosis is a parasitic disease that most frequently affects the central nervous system and is a major health problem in developing countries, with 50,000 deaths occurring every year. Neurocysticercosis-induced stroke is due to the inflammatory occlusion of small perforating arteries or deposits of atheromas in the arterial lumen. The hemorrhages are due to weakening of the arterial wall, with the formation of the mycotic aneurysms. Accurate diagnosis of neurocysticercosis is based on an assessment of clinical data in combination with the results of neuroimaging studies and immunologic tests.

gest that tea drinking is independently associated with prevalence of stroke and might play a role in the prevention of the disease.

India is ranked among the countries where the information on stroke is minimal. In a recent review of available information, the prevalence was estimated at 203 per 100,000 population. The estimation of stroke mortality was seriously limited by the method of classification of cause of death. Steps must be initiated to collect data on morbidity and mortality due to stroke in Asian countries as a first step toward implementing control measures.

CEREBROVASCULAR DISEASE IN THE TROPICS

Added to the presence of traditional risk factors for stroke, in the tropics, other nosologic entities that are prevalent in these regions constitute direct causes of stroke. Infectious or noninfectious conditions can be present: neurocysticercosis, malaria, sickle cell disease, tuberculosis, Chagas disease, viral hemorrhagic diseases (dengue fever), leptospirosis, snake bites, infective endocarditis, cerebral vein thrombosis, and others.

INFECTIOUS CONDITIONS

Neurocysticercosis Cysticercosis is the parasitic disease that most frequently affects the central nervous system and is one of the major health problems in nations of Latin America, Africa, and Asia. In endemic areas, neurocysticercosis (NCC) accounts for 10% of all hospital admissions to neurologic services. Almost 50,000 deaths due to NCC occur every year. Many more patients survive but are left with irreversible brain damage. NCC happens when humans incidentally become an intermediary host in the biologic cycle of *Taenia solium*, through ingesting eggs from contaminated water or food. The cysticercus can locate in the cerebral parenchyma, subarachnoid space, ventricular system, or spinal cord. Strokes are caused by the inflammatory occlusion of small perforating arteries in the base of the cranium or to the formation of deposits of atheroma in the arterial lumen. The hemorrhages, especially subarachnoid, result from the weakening of the arterial wall with formation of mycotic aneurysms.

Neurocysticercosis is a pleomorphic disease due to variations in the number and location of lesions. Focal signs may occur abruptly in patients who develop a cerebral infarct as a complication of subarachnoid NCC. Ischemic cerebrovascular complications of NCC include both lacunar and large cerebral infarcts. Lacunar infarcts are usually located in the posterior limb of the internal capsule or the corona radiata, and these infarcts produce typical lacunar syndromes (Case 1). Large cerebral infarcts are generally related to occlusion of the internal carotid artery or the anterior or middle cerebral artery. The accurate diagnosis of NCC is based on an assessment of the clinical data in combination with the results of neuroimaging studies and of immunologic tests. In patients with NCC-related stroke, computed tomography (CT) scan and magnetic resonance imaging (MRI) provide objective evidence of the topography of the infarct and demonstrate the characteristic features, including abnormal enhancement of the leptomeninges, hydrocephalus, and cystic lesions located usually at the sylvian fissure or basal cisterns. Cerebral angiography may demonstrate segmental narrowing or occlusion of intracranial arteries. Serologic tests are helpful, but should never be used alone to exclude or confirm the diagnosis; the most effective are immunoblots performed on serum and the CSF-ELISA test.

Therapy must be individualized according to the location of parasites and the degree of disease activity. Albendazole (15 mg/kg/d) for 8 days is advised for patients with viable subarachnoid cysts. Due to the proximity of subarachnoid cysts to the intracranial blood vessels, the inflammatory reaction that results from albendazole-related cyst destruction can enhance the process of occlusive endarteritis and thus the administration of steroids is mandatory.

Cerebral Malaria Malaria remains a serious public health problem in the tropics, mostly in Africa. Four *Plasmodium* species affect humans; of these, only *P. falciparum* invades the CNS, and it causes cerebral malaria. The infection is acquired when the parasite is inoculated across the skin from the bite of an Anopheles mosquito. Patients with cerebral malaria present with diffuse

CASE 1

A 39-year-old man, a farmer, with no medical history of diseases or hospitalizations, presents with a history of 2 years of recurrent headache with variable localization and intensity. These sometime last up to 1 week and get worse with exposure to cold, light, and noises and diminish with common analgesics. For the past 4 months, he notices progression in frequency and intensity of headache. He has stopped working. The headaches also are accompanied by deterioration of visual fields; vision is 'blurry' in both eyes, with a major problem in distant vision. He confuses colors, also day and night. Three weeks later, he begins to experience nausea and occasionally vomits gastric contents, sometimes three or four times a day. An ophthalmologist has ruled out ocular problems.

Four days ago, he suddenly presents with loss of strength in his left side and facial asymmetry. He says that his relatives couldn't understand him when he spoke. He denies sensitivity alterations, seizures, fever, or other symptoms. At evaluation, no venous pulse was present at funduscopy, he had left homonymous hemianopsia, and acute visual deterioration (20/400 in both eyes). He couldn't recognized blue and red from other colors. A left hemiparesis (+4/5) was noticed, with ipsilateral hyperreflexia, and Hoffman sign was positive. The rest of neurologic examination was normal. A CT scan and MRI evidenced multiple cysts and lesions mainly in the subarachnoid space, right sylvian fissure, and basal cisterns. Some of the lesions had perilesional edema. Secondary, a right basal ganglia compromise was observed, related to cerebral ischemic lacunar infarct (arrow), probably due to compression of the vascular structures by cysts. Angio-MRI did not show segmental narrowing or occlusion of intracranial arteries. Elisa for neurocysticercosis in CSF was positive 1:64. Immunoblot was not performed. Due to the risk of complications, he didn't receive albendazole, and it the disease managed with aspirin and corticosteroids.

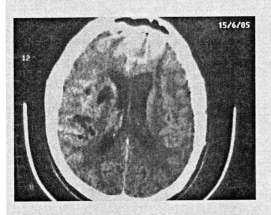
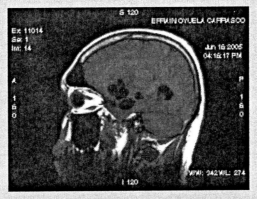
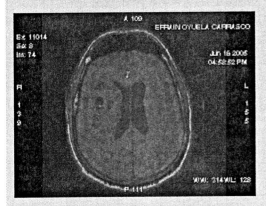
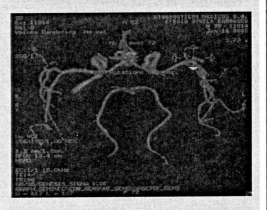

KEY POINTS

- Malaria remains a serious public health problem in the tropics, mostly in Africa. Of the four *Plasmodium* species, only *P. falciparum* invades the CNS and causes cerebral malaria. In cerebral malaria, either occlusion of cerebral capillaries or small subcortical hemorrhages can occur, due to vascular damage mediated by vasoactive substances. Despite therapy, up to 25% of patients die during the acute phase of cerebral malaria.

- Tuberculosis is an important cause of morbidity and mortality in tropical regions, with more than 8 million individuals infected every year. In tuberculosis, an inflammatory exudate invades the wall of arteries of small and medium caliber, with hyaline degeneration of the intimal layer, subendothelial cellular proliferation, and the presence of perivascular lymphocytes causing hemorrhages. Neuroimaging studies usually show hydrocephalus, abnormal enhancement of the basal leptomeninges, and cerebral infarcts. Antituberculous drugs must be given as soon as the diagnosis is suspected, since any delay is associated with increased mortality.

cerebral edema, small hemorrhages in subcortical white substance, and occlusion of cerebral capillaries by parasitic red cells. The hemorrhages result from the extravasation of erythrocytes due to the secondary vascular damage caused by a liberation of vasoactive substances. These findings suggest that cerebral damage in cerebral malaria is immunologic (humoral hypothesis of damage). The plugging of intracranial blood vessels is, however, related to an increased adherence of parasitized erythrocytes to the endothelium, with resulting brain damage due to obstruction of the cerebral microvasculature and reduced cerebral blood flow (mechanical hypothesis of damage). A combination of both, together with systemic complications of the disease, probably more satisfactorily explains the pathogenesis of cerebral malaria.

P. falciparum is identified by examination of blood smears using the Giemsa stain (Figure 4.1). Because parasitemia is cyclical, repeated examinations may be required. The CSF is normal in cerebral malaria. Neuroimaging studies may demonstrate brain swelling, cerebral infarcts, or small hemorrhages in severe cases. Quinine is the drug of choice for cerebral malaria, with an initial loading dose of 20 mg/kg infused over 4 hours, and a maintenance dose of 10 mg/kg every 8 to 12 hours, adjusted according to plasma concentrations. Corticosteroids

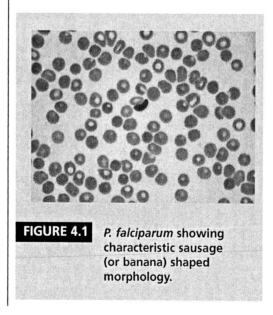

FIGURE 4.1 *P. falciparum* showing characteristic sausage (or banana) shaped morphology.

are harmful to comatose patients and should be avoided. Despite therapy, up to 25% of patients die during the acute phase of the disease.

Tuberculosis Tuberculosis is an important cause of morbidity and mortality in tropical regions, with more than 8 million individuals infected every year. The majority of the cases of tuberculosis is produced by infection with the bacillus *Mycobacterium tuberculosis*. This agent enters by the respiratory tract, where it establishes in the lungs and reaches the CNS by a hematogenous route. Once in cerebral parenchyma, the causal agent induces the development of an inflammatory response that ends with the formation of Rich's areas.

Among the histopathologic findings is an inflammatory exudate that invades the wall of arteries of small and medium caliber, with hyaline degeneration of the intimal layer, subendothelial cellular proliferation, and presence of perivascular lymphocytes. This degenerative process causes hemorrhages. The majority of these are located in the branched territories of the middle cerebral artery. They can be bilateral and symmetrical (Case 2). Massive strokes have been described that compromise the whole territory of the middle cerebral artery, as well as secondary events in the brainstem caused by the occlusion of the basilar artery. Intracranial hemorrhages are frequent. These can be related to the formation of mycotic aneurysms in patients with meningitis.

The CSF usually exhibits lymphocytic pleocytosis, increased protein, and low glucose content. Acid-fast bacilli are found in smears of CSF in a small percentage of cases. CSF cultures are positive in less than 50% of cases.

Neuroimaging studies usually show hydrocephalus, abnormal enhancement of the basal leptomeninges, and cerebral infarcts. The diagnosis of tuberculomas may be more difficult, because the imaged lesions may resemble other intracranial space-occupying lesions. Antituberculous drugs must be given as soon as the diagnosis is suspected, since any delay is associated with increased mortality. The mortality of patients with tuberculous meningoen-

CASE 2

A right-handed, 42-year-old woman with a history of tuberculosis detected 3 months ago (receiving treatment only for 8 weeks) comes to the emergency room with a history of sudden loss of strength of her left side, mostly in the face and arm. She has no cardiovascular risk factors. Through neurologic evaluation, a left motor deficit was found with signs of pyramidal dysfunction. CSF study showed pleocytosis with mononuclear predominance, elevated protein, and decrease of glucose, also with a positive adenosine deaminase study. CT scan revealed a vascular hypodensity in the right basal ganglia. This confirmed tubercular dissemination to the CNS, with secondary infectious vasculitis. Specific therapy was restarted using aspirin, with good clinical evolution. Two weeks later she was fully recovered from hemiparesis.

cephalitis who develop a stroke is three times greater than for patients who do not present this complication, and the survivors generally develop sequelae.

Chagas Disease Chagas disease (American trypanosomiasis) is a serious public health problem in South America, and it is becoming more important in developed nations due to a high flow of immigrants from endemic areas. This disease is caused by *Trypanosoma cruzi*, a protozoan that it is transmitted to humans through the bites of Triatominae insects. Up to 8% of the population in South America is seropositive, but only 10% to 30% of these develop symptomatic disease.

The cerebrovascular (CVD) complications appear in the chronic phase of the illness, and it is estimated that 9% to 36% of patients with chagasic myocardiopathy suffer CVD. Autopsy studies have detected left ventricular thrombi in one-third of patients who died from congestive heart failure or sudden death related to chronic Chagas disease. This is a major cardiac source of cerebral embolism. Due to the cardioembolic nature of the stroke, these usually are located in the territory of the middle cerebral artery and may produce hemorrhagic transformation (Case 3). Chagas disease can be diagnosed

by demonstration of *T. cruzi* in blood smears or CSF samples or by serologic testing. ECG abnormalities, such as left anterior fascicular block, right bundle-branch block, and atrial fibrillation, are common in patients with chronic disease but are not diagnostic. Neuroimaging usually demon-

CASE 3

A 42-year-old woman, right-handed, presented with a history of sudden loss of consciousness for approximately 30 minutes. She was found on the ground by relatives. When she reacted, they noticed that she did not mobilize the right side of her body and had difficulty speaking.

Two years ago, she was diagnosed with Chagas disease by a cardiologist, who did not indicate medical therapy because she presented to him in good condition, with normal vital signs.

Cardiomegaly and signs of aortic insufficiency were confirmed. Neurologically, she had a Glasgow Coma Scale 14/15, was confused, emotionally labile, dysarthric, and with a right hemiparesis, mostly in her arm, along with ipsilateral hypotonia, hyperreflexia, and Babinski sign. A CT scan done 6 days later revealed the presence of subacute vascular hypodensity, primarily at the left lenticular nuclei and corona radiata, suggestive of ischemic stroke. It was not possible to complete an echocardiographic examination. Due to Chagas disease, a cardioembolic mechanism was suspected, and low doses of warfarin were introduced. She had partial recovery of her neurologic deficit.

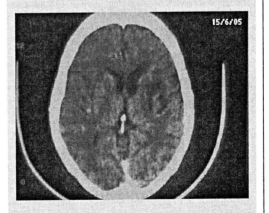

KEY POINTS

- Cerebro-vascular complications are observed in patients with cardiac arrhythmias or in those with cardiac insufficiency.

- Due to the cardioembolic nature of stroke, chronic treatment with oral anticoagulants is needed to avoid new events.

- Most cases of infective endocarditis (IE) are related to infections with *Streptococcus viridans* or *Staphylococcus aureus*. Cerebral infarcts in IE are related to the occlusion of cerebral arteries from embolic material derived from endocardial vegetations. They are most often located in the territory of the middle cerebral artery, and may have a hemorrhagic component. Patients require long-term anticoagulation therapy for primary and secondary stroke prevention.

- Leptospirosis is caused by *Leptospira interrogans*, and it is acquired after exposure of the skin and mucous membranes to water contaminated with this spirochete or by direct contact with the urine of infected animals. In leptospirosis, a large number of patients develop intracranial hemorrhages as a consequence of coagulopathy. Some patients also present with angiitis of intracranial vessels and should receive corticosteroids.

strates the location and extent of the cerebral infarct. Secondary prevention of stroke using long-term anticoagulation is recommended for all chagasic patients with stroke and heart failure, cardiac arrhythmias, or ventricular aneurysms.

Infective Endocarditis   Infective endocarditis (IE) is caused by colonization of the endocardium and heart valves by a variety of microorganisms, including, bacteria, rickettsiae, fungi, and chlamydia. Most cases are related to infections with *Streptococcus viridans* or *Staphylococcus aureus*. IE most commonly occurs in patients with prosthetic heart valves, and also in patients with predisposing conditions including rheumatic heart disease, congenital heart disease, open heart surgery, mitral valve prolapse, hemodialysis, and intravenous drug abuse. IE is a common cause of neurologic disability in developing countries, particularly in those in which rheumatic heart disease is still prevalent.

Patients may develop a variety of neurologic complications, including, meningitis, brain abscesses, and ischemic or hemorrhage strokes. Cerebral infarcts in IE are related to the occlusion of cerebral arteries from embolic material derived from endocardial vegetations. They are most often located in the territory of the middle cerebral artery, and may have a hemorrhagic component, particularly in patients receiving anticoagulants. Intracranial hemorrhages may be related to acute necrotizing arteritis or to the rupture of a mycotic aneurysm.

IE should be suspected in patients with heart murmur and fever, particularly if a pre-existing heart disease or another predisposing condition is present. Blood cultures identify the etiologic agent in up to 85% of cases. Echocardiography allows the visualization of vegetations and other cardiac lesions. Antibiotics must be given to all patients with suspected IE, to eradicate the causal microorganisms. Surgical valve replacement plays an important role in management. Patients require long-term anticoagulation therapy for primary and secondary stroke prevention.

Leptospirosis   This disease is rare in developed countries but represents a common health problem in tropical areas of

Southeast Asia and Latin America. Leptospirosis is caused by *Leptospira interrogans* and is acquired generally after exposure of the skin and mucosa to water contaminated with this spirochete or by direct contact with the urine of infected animals (rats, dogs, etc.). The toxic effects of this infection induce, along with other complications, acute tubular necrosis, coagulopathies secondary to vasculitis, myocarditis, meningitis, and uveitis. The neurologic disease limits itself generally to aseptic meningitis, which can progress, in some cases, toward an encephalitis. A large number of patients also develop intracranial hemorrhages as a consequence of coagulopathy. Some patients present angiitis of intracranial vessels, which can determine the development of a net of collateral vessels similar to that observed in moyamoya disease. In fact, some authors consider that leptospirosis is a cause of moyamoya disease in China and other countries of Asia.

Diagnosis should be confirmed by isolation of *L. interrogans* in blood or urine cultures or by demonstration of a fourfold rise in the titers of specific antibodies. A CT scan and MRI are useful in demonstrating the presence of cerebrovascular complications of the disease, both intracranial hemorrhages and cerebral infarcts. Angiography may show the development of a rich network of collaterals. Penicillin or doxycycline for 1 week are useful against the pathogen. Patients with angiitis should receive corticosteroids.

Viral Hemorrhagic Diseases   Viral hemorrhagic fever includes a series of entities capable of producing, among other manifestations, intracranial hemorrhage. These diseases involve thousands of individuals in the tropics. They appear in the form of epidemic outbreaks confined to different geographic regions, and they can be transmitted by vectors (mosquitos, ticks) or by person-to-person contact (Table 4.3).

The mechanisms that favor the development of a hemorrhage include an increase in vascular permeability, platelet function alteration, thrombocytopenia, and disseminated intravascular coagulation. Patients usually present with fever, headache, muscle pain, and multiple sites of bleeding. When the disease progresses to compromising the CNS, there is frequent development of acute encephalitis, with delirium, deterioration of consciousness, and convulsive crisis. It is rare to observe focal signs, despite the fact that many patients with viral fevers present with hemorrhages in cerebral tissue or in the subarachnoid space. Virus isolation or detection of specific antibodies in serum permits the correct diagnosis. Supportive measures and a correction of coagulation problems are the cornerstones of therapy for most viral hemorrhagic fever.

NONINFECTIOUS CONDITIONS

Snake Bites Poisonous snakes represent a health problem for people who live in rural areas of the tropics. For example, snake bites are responsible for up to 20% of deaths in inhabitants of some Amazonian tribes, and they are a cause of more than 20,000 deaths per year in Asia. Snake venom is probably the most complex of all known poisons. It contains, among other components, phospholipase A2, acetylcholinesterase, hyaluronidase, metalloproteinases, and serine proteases. Some of these enzymes have a direct neurotoxic effect, whereas others induce cerebrovascular events by procoagulant or fibrinolytic activity. The probable reasons of secondary CVD are vascular hemolysis, disseminated intravascular coagulation, toxic vasculitis, and hypovolemic shock. Some patients present with neurologic focal signs secondary to the development of a cerebral hemorrhage (Case 4).

Neuroimaging studies allow the proper recognition of the cerebrovascular complications of snakebites. The hemorrhages can be located in any part of cerebral parenchyma or in the subarachnoid space; usually multiple hemorrhages are present, located in different arterial territories. Those patients with hemorrhages have an elevation of products of fibrinogen degradation and also an alteration in coagulation times. Polyspecific antivenom and supportive measures are the cornerstone of therapy. In patients with intracranial hemorrhages, the reintroduction of fresh plasma and the use of vitamin K is recommended and, in those with stroke, the use of corticosteroids is indicated.

KEY POINTS

- Viral hemorrhagic fevers are a series of entities capable of producing, among other manifestations, intracranial hemorrhage. The mechanisms that favor the development of a hemorrhage include an increase in the vascular permeability, platelet function alteration, thrombocytopenia, and disseminated intravascular coagulation. Supportive measures and correction of coagulation problems are the cornerstones of therapy for most viral hemorrhagic fevers.

- In snake bites, the causes of secondary CVD are vascular hemolysis, disseminated intravascular coagulation, toxic vasculitis, and hypovolemic shock. These hemorrhages can be located in any part of cerebral parenchyma or in the subarachnoid space; usually they are multiple and located in different arterial territories. Polyspecific antivenom and supportive measures are the cornerstones of snake-bite therapy.

TABLE 4.3 **Viral Hemorrhagic Fevers**

Disease	Etiology/Transmission	Geographic Distribution
Argentian hemorrhagic fever	Jurin viruses Rats to humans	Argentina
Bolivian hemorrhagic fever	Machupo viruses Rats to humans	Bolivia
Crimean-Congo hemorrhagic fever	Crimean-Congo viruses Ticks to humans	Africa, Eastern Europe, Middle East, China
Hemorrhagic Dengue fever	Dengue viruses Mosquitos to humans	Latin American, Asia, Africa
Ebola	Ebola virus Primates to humans	Central Africa
Hantavirus diseases	Hantavirus Rats to humans	Worldwide
Kyasanur disease	Flaviviruses Ticks to humans	India
Yellow fever	Flaviviruses Mosquitos to humans	South America, Africa

Reproduced and translated with permission from: O.H. del Brutto. Enfermedad cerebrovascular en los trópicos. *Rev Neurol* 2001; 33:750–62.

KEY POINTS

- Thrombosis of the cerebral veins and sinuses is a distinct cerebrovascular disorder that, unlike arterial stroke, most often affects young adults and children.

- A prothrombotic risk factor or a direct cause is identified in about 85% of patients with sinus thrombosis. The clinical presentation is highly variable, and anticoagulation is the most obvious treatment option available.

- Sickle cell disease results in a loss of red cell deformability, which causes the occlusion of small vessels and favors cerebral ischemia. Every year it affects more than 100,000 children born in Africa, of which only 5% will survive up to school age.

- Approximately 15% of sickle cell disease patients present with CVD, which can be ischemic or hemorrhagic, with events of different size and location. These CVDs are related to diverse etiopathogenic mechanisms.

CASE 4

A 39-year-old man, married, presents to the emergency room with a history of snake-bite from a Cascavel (*Crotalus durissus*) in his right foot. Thirty minutes after the bite, he presented gingivorrhage, aphasia, syncope, and gastrointestinal bleeding. The neurologic examination demonstrated a Glasgow Coma Scale of 14 and confused speech. Funduscopy did not reveal papilledema. A left-sided hemiparesis and left Babinski sign were detected, with normal sensibility and absence of meningeal signs. In addition, he presented equimosis in his tongue and right leg. Five days later, he had neck rigidity, with a Glasgow score of 13/15, and developed right hemiparesis and a bilateral Babinski sign. Neurologic deterioration led to his death.

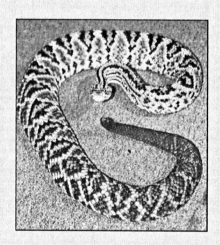

Cerebral Vein Thrombosis Thrombosis of the cerebral veins and sinuses is a distinct cerebrovascular disorder that, unlike arterial stroke, most often affects young adults and children. About 75% of the adult patients are women. It represents one of the most important causes of stroke in women of reproductive age living in Asia and Latin America. A prothrombotic risk factor or a direct cause is identified in about 85% of patients with sinus thrombosis, including genetic prothrombotic conditions, pregnancy, puerperium, cranial infections, systemic inflammatory diseases, hematologic conditions, medications, cancer, and others. The clinical presentation is highly variable; CT scan and MRI may show unilateral or bilateral infarcts, hemorrhagic or non-hemorrhagic, in up to 50% of patients (Case 5). Angiography usually shows total or partial occlusion of one or more of the dural sinuses or cerebral veins. Presently, anticoagulation is the most obvious treatment option available.

Sickle Cell Disease Sickle cell disease is genetically determined and is recessively inherited from two abnormal genes, one of which is the gene for sickle cells, responsible for the synthesis of beta chains in the hemoglobin. It is prevalent in Africa, especially in areas where cerebral malaria is endemic. Indeed, the sickle cell gene appeared as a mutation during human evolution, inducing changes in hemoglobin that render the erythrocyte less susceptible to malarial infection. Every year, it affects more than 100,000 children born in Africa, of which only 5% will survive up to school age. The anomalous structure of the hemoglobin impedes normal oxygen transportation to the tissues and also affects red cell deformability, which in turn determines the occlusion of small blood vessels and favors the development of ischemia. Approximately 15 % of patients present with CVD, which can be ischemic or hemorrhagic, with events of different size and location related to diverse etiopathogenic mechanisms. Strokes can be precipitated by episodes of acidosis, infections, or a sudden fall in the concentration of hemoglobin. Protein electrophoresis permits the correct diagnosis. No evidence suggests that antiplatelet agents or anticoagulants are of value for stroke management in these patients.

Acknowledgment
We would like to acknowledge Drs. FJ Carod-Artal, Reyna Duron, and Oscar del Brutto. This paper was supported by an educational grant from the Honduras Neurology Training Program and the Sociedad Española de Neurologia.

CASE 5

A 29-year-old woman presents with a history of 2 months of universal, daily, pulsatile headache of moderate intensity that attenuates only with injected analgesics, along with nausea and occasional vomiting. She has decreased strength and drift of her left arm; she is unable to articulate words, so her relatives decided to bring her to the hospital. She denied fever, seizures, blurry vision, or medications. Her past medical history was completely normal. On examination, vital signs were normal, but she had bilateral papilledema and monoparesis—4/5 in her left arm. The rest of the neurologic examination was normal.

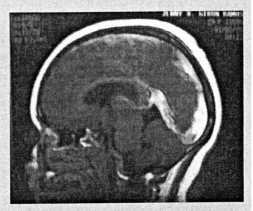

She was hospitalized, and a lumbar puncture revealed an opening pressure of 28 cm H_2O. The CSF analysis was normal. The MRI showed a hyperintense signal in T1, T2, and FLAIR sequences that crossed along the superior sagittal sinus (see figure). The image strongly suggested venous sinus thrombosis. Secondarily, a slight ventricular expansion toward the third ventricle was observed, which caused compression on the optical chiasma. A widespread inflammatory process compressed the subarachnoid spaces. Antiphospholipid autoantibodies were positive. The patient was anticoagulated initially with unfractionated heparin and had a full recovery. She was discharged with warfarin, and a 2.5 INR was obtained. Follow-up at 3 months did not show neurologic complication or bleeding.

REFERENCES

Aho K, Harmsen P, Hatano S, Marquardsen J, Smirnov VE, Strasser T. Cerebrovascular disease in the community: results of a WHO collaborative study. *Bull World Health Organ* 1980;58:113–130.

Barinagarrementeria F, Cantú C, Arredonto H. Aseptic cerebral venous thrombosis: proposed prognostic scale. *J Stroke Cerebrovasc Dis* 1992; 2: 34–39. (Manifestations associated with poor prognosis in patients with puerperal venous thrombosis include stupor or coma, bilateral pyramidal tract signs, generalized seizures, meningeal signs, bilateral lesions on CT scans, and hemorrhagic cerebrospinal fluid.)

Bonita R, Mendis S, Truelsen T, et al. The Global Stroke Initiative. *Lancet Neurology* 2004;3:391–93. (A stepwise approach to increasing detail in the data to be collected for surveillance of stroke is suggested, to allow countries with different levels of resources and capacity in their health systems to collect useful information for policy.)

Bonita R, Stewart A, Beaglehole R. International trends in stroke mortality: 1970–1985. *Stroke* 1990;21:989–92. (This study compared the pattern of cerebrovascular disease (stroke) mortality in men and women aged 40 to 69 years in 27 countries during 1970–1985 with the decline in coronary heart disease mortality during the same period.)

Brainin M, Bornstein N, Boysen G, Demarin V. Acute neurologic stroke care in Europe: Results of the European Stroke Care Inventory. *Eur J Neurol* 2000;7:5–10. (A European inventory was undertaken to assess the development of acute stroke care in European countries and to give an estimate of the needs, based on 1997 data. Information from 22 countries was based either on national surveys, hospital statistics, or estimates given on the basis of extrapolation of regional studies, or other defined sources.)

Cantu C, Barinagarrementeria F. Cerebrovascular complications of neurocysticercosis. Clinical and neuroimaging spectrum. *Arch Neurol* 1996;53(3):233–39. (This article describes the clinical and neuroimaging spectrum of cerebral cysticercus arteritis and clarifies the mechanisms of a stroke associated with neurocysticercosis, describing a number of cases from a tertiary-care center.)

Carod-Artal FJ, Vargas AP, Melo M, Horan TA. American trypanosomiasis (Chagas disease): an unrecognized cause of stroke. *J Neurol Neurosurg Psychiatry* 2003;74(4):516–18.

Del Brutto. Enfermedad cerebrovascular en los trópicos. *Rev Neurol* 2001;33:750–62. (A review of the clinical manifestations, diagnosis, and therapy of diseases causing cerebrovascular disease in the tropics.)

Feigin VL, Lawes CMM, Bennett DA, Anderson CS. Stroke epidemiology: a review of population-based studies of incidence, prevalence, and case-fatality in the late 20th century. *Lancet Neurology* 2003;2:43–53. (An overview of population-based studies of incidence, prevalence, mortality, and case-fatality of stroke based on studies from 1990.)

Hsieh F-Y, Chia L-G, Shen W-C. Location of cerebral infarctions in tuberculous meningitis. *Neuroradiology* 1992;34:197–99. (The locations of cerebral infarctions is studied in 14 patients with tuberculous meningitis [TBM]. 75% of infarctions occurred in the "TB zone" supplied by medial striate and thalamoperforating arteries.)

Ibidapo MO, Akinyanju OO. Acute sickle cell syndromes in Nigerian adults. *Clin Lab Haematol* 2000;22:151–55. (In this study, the pattern of acute illness was determined in 102 adolescents and adults with sickle cell anemia who presented to the emergency unit of a Lagos hospital, in Nigeria.)

Kaste M, Fogelholm R, Rissanen A. Economic burden of stroke and the development of new therapies. *Public Health* 1998 Mar;112(2):103–12. (A review of the costs of stroke in developed and developing countries; also discusses stroke measures of functional outcome, as a primary endpoint in stroke trials.)

Kesteloot H, Sans S, Kromhout D. Evolution of all-causes and cardiovascular mortality in the age-group 75–84 years in Europe during the period 1970–1996; a comparison with worldwide changes. *Eur Heart J* 2002 Mar;23(5):384–98.

Lessa I, Cortes E. Cerebrovascular accident as a complication of leptospirosis. *Lancet* 1981;2:1113.

Mosquera A, Idrovo LA, Tafur A, Del Brutto OH. Stroke following *Bothrops* spp. snakebite. *Neurology* 2003;60(10):1577–80. (A review of 309 consecutive patients bitten by *Bothrops* spp. who were attended at a large general hospital. The prevalence of cerebrovascular complications related to *Bothrops* spp. bites was 2.6%.)

Murray CJL, López AD. Alternative projections of mortality and disability by cause, 1990–2020: Global Burden of Disease Study. *Lancet* 1997;349:1498–504.

Newton CR, Hien TT, White N. Cerebral malaria. *J Neurol Neurosurg Psychiatry* 2000;69:433–41.(A review of the different pathogeneses and clinical presentations of cerebral malaria between adults and children.)

Poungvarin N. Stroke in the developing world. *Lancet* 1998;352(Suppl III):19–22.

Saposnik G, Del Brutto OH. Stroke in South America: a systematic review of incidence, prevalence, and stroke subtypes. *Stroke* 2003 Sep;34(9):2103–7. (A systematic review of articles on stroke in South America, with emphasis on those providing information on the incidence and prevalence of stroke [community-based studies] and the pattern of stroke subtypes [hospital-based studies].

Sarti E, Rastenyte D, Cepaitis Z, Tuomilehto J. International trends in mortality from stroke 1968 to 1994. *Stroke* 2000;31:1588–1601. (This study present rates and trends in mortality from stroke up to 1994. Data are presented for men and women in 51 industrialized and developing countries from different parts of the world. They observed large differences in mortality rates from stroke around the world, with a wide variation in mortality trends.)

Téllez-Zenteno JF, Negrete-Pulido O, Cantu C, et al. Hemorrhagic stroke associated to neurocysticercosis. *Neurologia* 2003;18(5):272–75. (A report of two cases with this association; cerebral hemorrhages were considered to be related to cysticercotic arteritis of small penetrating vessels.)

WHO MONICA Project (prepared by Thorvaldsen P, Kuulasmaa K, Rajakangas A-M, Rastenyte D, Sarti C, Wilhelmsen L). Stroke trends in the WHO MONICA Project. *Stroke* 1997;28:500–6. (Stroke registries were established as part of the international collaborative World Health Organization Monitoring of Trends and Determinants in Cardiovascular Disease [WHO MONICA] Project in 17 centers in 10 countries. The aim of the present analyses was to estimate and compare temporal stroke trends across the MONICA populations.)

Wolf PA, D'Agnostino RB, Belanger AJ, Kannel WB. Probability of stroke: a risk profile from the Framingham Study. *Stroke* 1991;22:312–18. (The authors sought to modify existing sex-specific health risk appraisal functions [profile functions] for the prediction of first stroke to better assess the effects of the use of antihypertensive medication.)

World Health Organization / World Federation of Neurology. *Atlas: Country Resources for Neurologic Diseases 2004.* Geneva: WHO, 2004. (Project Atlas was launched by the WHO in 2000, with the object of collecting, compiling, and disseminating relevant information in the area of neurology and neurologic services in different countries. All data were collected from a large international study carried out in 2001–2003, which included 109 countries spanning all six WHO regions and covering over 90% of the world population.)

INDEX

activities of daily living (ADLs), 37, 41, 42
activity at onset of stroke, 15–16
acute disseminated encephomyelitis (ADEM), 21
affective disorders, 43–45
Africa and stroke, 53, 54
Agency for Health Care Policy and Research (AHCPR), 34
albendazole, 54
alcohol consumption, 50, 52
amphetamines and stroke, 15
aneurysm, 6, 15, 18
animal experiments, 27
anticoagulation therapy, 40
antithrombin time, 25
aphasia, 32
apraxia, 32
Argentina, 52
arthritis, 34
Asia and stroke, 53–54
ataxia, 32
atheromatous brachial disease, 12, 17
atherosclerosis, 12–13, 14
Australia, 2, 3

balance difficulties, 16
Barthel index, 37
bladder control, 40
blood pressure and stroke, 14–16, 41, 52. *See also* hypertension
bowel control, 41
brain ischemia, 11–13. *See also* ischemic stroke
   blood tests and, 25
   imaging studies and, 23–25
brain tumors, 21
brainstem infarcts, 23
burden of stroke, 1–2

calcium metabolism, 25
Canada, 2
cardioembolic stroke, 6
cardiovascular/heart disease, 15, 16, 34, 52, 53
Caribbean and stroke, 52–53
carotid artery, 16, 17

carotid endarterectomy, 40
Cascavel (*Crotalus durissus*), **60**
cerebellar arteries, 17
cerebellar infarcts, 23
cerebral arteries, 17
cerebral infarction, 6
cerebral venous thrombosis, 52*t*, 60
cerebrovascular disease, 49
Chagas disease, 52, 52*t*, 57–58, **57**
China, 53–54
cholesterol, 25
classification of stroke, 6
clinical course, 15
coagulation factors, 25
cocaine and stroke, 15, 22
cognitive dysfunction, 43
communication. *See* language and communication
comorbid disease processes and stroke, **35**
compensation in recovery, 32–33
complex regional pain syndrome (CRPS), 42, **42**
computed tomography (CT), 21–25
cortical infarcts, 23
cost of stroke, 2
Crotalus durissus (Cascavel), **60**
CT angiography (CTA), 21–25
Cuba, 52
cysticercosis, 54–55, **55**
cytomegalovirus (CMV), 21
Czechoslovakia, 2

deep venous thrombosis (DVT), 40
depression, long-term (LTD), 29
developing countries and stroke, 49–62. *See also* infectious causes of stroke; noninfectious causes of stroke
   Africa and, 53
   Asia and the Middle East, 53–54
   Caribbean and, 52–53
   Eastern Europe and, 53
   international trends in epidemiology of, 50, 51*t*
   Latin America and, 50–52, 51*t*
   populations of, 49–50

developing countries and stroke (*continued*)
   risk factors and, 50
   smoking and, 50
diabetes, 14, 34, 40, 50, 52
diagnosis, 18–25
diaschisis and recovery, 31–32
diet, 50, 53
differential diagnosis, 21
diffusion-weighted MRI (DWI), 25
disability-adjusted life years (DALYs) and stroke, 1, 1*t*, 2*t*
donepezil, 44
dysarthria, 43. *See also* language and communications
dysphagia, 40

Eastern Europe and stroke, 53
echocardiography, 21, 24
ecology of stroke, 14–16
Ecuador, 52
electroencephalograms (EEGs), 25
embolism, 6, 12, 13
   imaging studies and, 23–24
   location of vascular pathology in, 1
endocarditis, infective (IE), 52*t*, 58
epidemiology of stroke, 1–8
   international trends in, 50, 51*t*
epilepsy, 49
eye examination, 16

Factors VII/VIII, 25
falls, 41–43
family history of stroke, 14
fever, 16
fibrinogens, 25
Finland, 34
flaccidity, 42
fluid-attenuated inversion recovery (FLAIR), 22
France, 3, 7
Frenchay Health District Stroke Registry, 34
functional assessment and outcome measurement of stroke survivors, 34, 36–38

functional deficits in stroke, **35**
functional imaging, 28–29
Functional Independence Measurement
        (FIM), 37, 37*t*
functional magnetic resonance imaging
        (fMRI), 28–29

GABA-B, 33
gender differences in stroke, 14, 34
genetic testing, 25

headache, 16, 20
heart disease. *See* cardiovascular disease
hemorrhage, 15–16
hemorrhagic fevers (viral), 52*t*, 58–59, 59*t*
hemorrhagic stroke, 9
        imaging studies for, 22
heparin, 40
herpes zoster varicella (HZV), 21
heterogeneity of stroke, 5–6
high-intensity transient signals (HITS), 24
history, 14–16
HIV/AIDS, 25, 53
hyperlipidemia, 14
hypertension, 14, 15, 40, 50, 53. *See also*
        blood pressure

Ibero-American Societies of Neurology, 50
imaging studies, 21–25
        brain ischemia and, 23–25
        Chagas disease in, 57–58, **57**
        embolism and, 23–24
        functional, 28–29
        infarcts and, 23–25
        intracerebral hemorrhage and, 22
        ischemic vs. hemorrhagic lesions in, 22
        malaria and Plasmodium in, 56, **56**
        neurocysticercosis, 54–55, **55**
        occlusive disease and, 23–24
        SAH and, 23
        snake bites and, 59–60
        tuberculosis, 56–57
incidence of stroke, 3–5, 4, **5**
independent ADLs (IADLs), 37
India, 54
infarcts, 23–25
infectious causes of stroke, 52*t*, 54–59
intercerebral hemorrhage, location of vas-
        cular pathology in 17–18
interdisciplinary units (stroke units) in, 45,
        46*t*
International Classification of Functioning,
        Disability and Health (ICIDH), 36,
        36*t*
intracerebral hemorrhage (ICH), 5–6,
        9–10, 15, 16
        imaging studies and, 22
intracranial hemorrhage, 9–11

ischemic stroke, 6, 9, 11–13
        imaging studies for, 22

L-dopa, 44
laboratory tests, 21, 25
lacunar infarction, 6, 23
language and communication, 16–17, 37,
        43
Latin America and stroke, 50–52, 51*t*, 54
leading causes of death, 1, 1%
learned non-use, 31
leptospirosis, *Leptospira interrogans*, 52*t*,
        58
life expectancy after stroke, 1–2
lipid panels, 25
lipohyalinosis, 12, 17
locations of vascular pathologies, 17–18
low-molecular-weight heparin (LMWH),
        40
Lyme disease, 25

magnetic resonance angiography (MRA),
        21–25
magnetic resonance imaging (MRI),
        21–25, 28–29, 33
magnetic stimulation. *See* transcranial
        magnetic stimulation (TMS)
malaria, 52, 52*t*, 56, **56**, 60
Martinique, 52
memory, 43
Mexico, 52
Middle East and stroke, 53–54
migraine, 20
mobilization, 41–43
Monitoring Trends and Determinants in
        Cardiovascular Disease (MONICA),
        5, 53
mortality and stroke, 2–3, 3, **4**, 49
motor evoked potential (MEP), 29
motor signs, 16–17
Mycobacterium tuberculosis, 56

National Clinical Guidelines, 45
National Institute of Health Stroke Scale
        (NIHSS), 41
neurocysticercosis, 52, 52*t*, 54–55, **55**
neurologic findings, 16–17
neuropsychological alteration, 43–45
neurorehabilitation, 33–45
New Zealand, 5
noninfectious causes of stroke, 52*t*, 59–60
nonketotic hyperglycemic stupor, 21
North East Melbourne Stroke Incidence
        Study (NEMESIS), 2, 3–4

obesity, 34
occlusive disease, 23–24
orthostatic reactions, 41

outcome of stroke, 6, 34, 34*t*, 35*t*, 36*t*
Oxfordshire Community Stroke Study, 6

pain, 42, **42**
parenchymal hemorrhage, 9. *See also*
        intracerebral hemorrhage (ICH)
pathogenesis of stroke, 6
penumbra, 33
People's Republic of China, 53–54
perceptual deficits and unilateral neglect,
        43
perfusion-weighted MRI (PWI), 25
perilesional area role in recovery, 33
psychosocial functioning, 43
physical examination, 16–17
Plasmodium falciparum, 52, 56, **56**
plasticity of brain in recovery, 27–28, 29
Portugal, 2
positron emission tomography (PET), 25,
        28
post-stroke depression (PSD), 43
Post-Stroke Rehabilitation Guideline
        Panel, 43
potentiation, long-term (LTP), 29
prediction factors of functional outcome,
        34, 34*t*, 35*t*, 36*t*
prevalence of stroke, 5, 49, 50
preventing stroke, 6–7, 39
professional context factors in recovery,
        45
PROGRESS study, 6
protein C, 25
prothrombin, 25
psychosocial functioning, 37
pulmonary embolism (PE), 40
pulse, 16
pure motor stroke, 16

racial differences in stroke, 14
Rankin scale, 37
reafferent feedback, 29–33
recovery and rehabilitation, 27–47
        analysis of, 31, **32**
        Barthel index for, 37
        bladder control and, 40
        comorbid disease processes and, **35**
        compensation in, 32–33
        diaschisis and, 31–32
        dysphagia and, 40
        functional assessment and outcome
                measurement of stroke survivors in,
                34, 36–38
        functional deficits in, **35**
        functional imaging and, 28–29
        Functional Independence Measurement
                (FIM) for, 37, 37*t*
        interdisciplinary units (stroke units) in,
                45, 46*t*

recovery and rehabilitation (*continued*)
  learned non-use and, 31
  mechanisms of, 27–33
  neuropsychological alteration and, 43
  neurorehabilitation in, 33–45
  perceptual deficits and unilateral
    neglect in, 43
  perilesional area role in, 33
  plasticity of brain and, 27–28, 29
  prediction factors of functional out-
    come in, 34, 34*t*, 35*t*, 36*t*
  prevention of recurrence and, 39
  process of, and techniques used in, 39
  programs for, 34–40
  progress monitoring in, 37
  Rankin scale for, 37
  reafferent feedback in, 29–33
  reorganization of brain in, 28–29
  sensorimotor, 41–43
  setting of programs for, 38–39, **39**
  social and professional context factors
    in, 43
  transcranial magnetic stimulation
    (TMS) and, 29
  U.S. Agency for Health Care Policy
    and Research guidelines for, 45,
    46*t*
  visual system role in, 31
  WHO definition of, 33
recurrence of stroke, 6
regional cerebral bloodflow (RCBF), 28
reorganization of brain in recovery, 28–29
risk factors for stroke, 6, 14–16, 50
Russia, 3, 5, 53

Scottish Guidelines, 45
seizures, 16, 20
sensorimotor rehabilitation, 41–43
sentinel leaks, 16
settings for recovery, 38–39, **39**
sexual functioning, 37

shoulder problems, 42
sickle cell disease, 52*t*, 60
Singapore, 53
single photon emission computed tomography (SPECT), 25
skin protection, 40, 42
smoking and stroke, 14–16, 40, 50, 52
snake bites, 52, 52*t*, 59–60
social and professional context factors in
  recovery, 43
somatosensory evoked potentials (SSEPs),
  30
spasticity, 41
Staphylococcus aureus, 58
Streptococcus viridians, 58
stroke units, 45
subarachnoid hemorrhage (SAH), 6, 9,
  10–11, 15, 16
  imaging studies and, 22, 23
  location of vascular pathology in, 18
subcortical infarcts, 23
subhyaloid hemorrhage, 16
subtypes of stroke, 9–26
survival, 36
swallowing. *See* dysphagia
Sweden, 5
symptoms, 16
synapses
  intensive stimulation and structural
    changes of, 11, **31**
  plasticity of, 29, **30**
  structural changes of, **10**
syphilis, 25
systemic hypoperfusion, 12, 13

Taenia solium, 54
Tanzania, 53
temporal arteritis, 17
thrombosis, 11, 12–13, 15, 16, 60
  location of vascular pathology in, 17
TOAST system, 6

tobacco use, 50. *See also* smoking
transcranial magnetic stimulation (TMS),
  29
transcranial Doppler ultrasound (TCD),
  23, 24–25
transient ischemic attacks (TIAs), 14, 15,
  40
  diagnosis of, 18–21, 19%
  differential diagnosis for, 19%
  seizures and, 20
transthoracic echocardiography (TTE), 24
trauma and stroke, 15–16
Trypanosoma cruzi, 57–58
tuberculosis, 52*t*, 56–57
tumors, 21

U.S. Agency for Health Care Policy and
  Research guidelines, 45, 46*t*
U.S. Center for Disease Control (CDC), 50
ultrasound, 21, 23, 24–25
unilateral neglect, 43
United States, 2, 4, 5, 7
Urinary Incontinence in Adults, 40. *See
  also* bladder control

vascular malformations, 18
vertebral arteries, 17
video fluoroscopy/endoscopy, 40
viral infection, 21. *See also* hemorrhagic
  fevers
visual system role in recovery, 31
vomiting, 16, 20
von Willebrand factor, 25

walking (ambulation), 36, 41–43
World Bank, burden of stroke and, 1–2
World Health Organization (WHO), 49
  rehabilitation defined by, 33

xenon-enhanced CT, 25